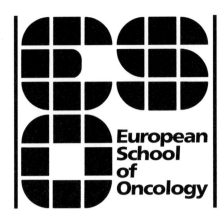

European School of Oncology

Monographs
Series Editor: U. Veronesi

The European School of Oncology gratefully acknowledges the educational grant for the production of this monograph received from GE Medical Systems and Kodak SpA Italy

A. Gad   M. Rosselli Del Turco (Eds.)

Breast Cancer Screening in Europe

With 25 Figures and 39 Tables

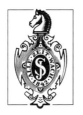

Springer-Verlag
Berlin Heidelberg New York
London Paris Tokyo
Hong Kong Barcelona
Budapest

ADEL GAD, M.D., Ph.D., Associate Professor

Department of Clinical Pathology and Cytology
Falun Hospital
791 82 Falun, Sweden

MARCO ROSSELLI DEL TURCO, M.D.

Centro per lo Studio e la
Prevenzione Oncologica
Viale A. Volta, 171
50131 Firenze, Italy

ISBN 3-540-56577-9 Springer-Verlag Berlin Heidelberg New York
ISBN 0-387-56577-9 Springer-Verlag New York Berlin Heidelberg

Library of Congress Cataloging-in-Publication Data
Breast cancer screening in Europe / A. Gad, M. Rosselli Del Turco (eds.).
  (Monographs / European School of Oncology)
Includes bibliographical references.
  ISBN 3-540-56577-9 (alk. paper)
  ISBN 0-387-56577-9 (alk. paper)
1. Breast–Cancer–Europe. 2. Medical screening–Europe. I. Gad, Adel. II. Rosselli Del Turco, M. (Marco), 1948- . III.
Series: Monographs (European School of Oncology) [DNLM: 1. Breast Neoplasms–prevention & control–Europe. 2.
Mass Screening. WP 870 B82842 1993] RC280.B8B6847 1993 362.1'9699449'0094–dc20 DNLM/DLC for Library of
Congress

Typesetting: Camera ready by editor
Printing: Druckhaus Beltz, Hemsbach/Bergstr.; Binding: J. Schäffer GmbH & Co. KG, Grünstadt
23/3145 - 5 4 3 2 1 0 – Printed on acid-free paper

Foreword

The European School of Oncology came into existence to respond to a need for information, education and training in the field of the diagnosis and treatment of cancer. There are two main reasons why such an initiative was considered necessary. Firstly, the teaching of oncology requires a rigorously multidisciplinary approach which is difficult for the Universities to put into practice since their system is mainly disciplinary orientated. Secondly, the rate of technological development that impinges on the diagnosis and treatment of cancer has been so rapid that it is not an easy task for medical faculties to adapt their curricula flexibly.

With its residential courses for organ pathologies and the seminars on new techniques (laser, monoclonal antibodies, imaging techniques etc.) or on the principal therapeutic controversies (conservative or mutilating surgery, primary or adjuvant chemotherapy, radiotherapy alone or integrated), it is the ambition of the European School of Oncology to fill a cultural and scientific gap and, thereby, create a bridge between the University and Industry and between these two and daily medical practice.

One of the more recent initiatives of ESO has been the institution of permanent study groups, also called task forces, where a limited number of leading experts are invited to meet once a year with the aim of defining the state of the art and possibly reaching a consensus on future developments in specific fields of oncology.

The ESO Monograph series was designed with the specific purpose of disseminating the results of these study group meetings, and providing concise and updated reviews of the topic discussed.

It was decided to keep the layout relatively simple, in order to restrict the costs and make the monographs available in the shortest possible time, thus overcoming a common problem in medical literature: that of the material being outdated even before publication.

UMBERTO VERONESI
Chairman Scientific Committee
European School of Oncology

Contents

Introduction
A. GAD and M. ROSSELLI DEL TURCO 1

Breast Cancer: The Scene in Europe
F. DE WAARD 3

Overview of European Screening Programmes
L. PAS and B.-P. ROBRA 7

Evidence of the Effectiveness of Breast Cancer Screening
J. CHAMBERLAIN and D. PALLI 15

Cost-Effectiveness Analysis of Breast Cancer Screening
H. J. DE KONING, J. D. F. HABBEMA, B. M. VAN INEVELD and G. J. VAN OORTMARSSEN 25

Programme Organisation in Breast Cancer Screening
B. A. THOMAS 35

Compliance in Breast Cancer Screening: the Spanish Experience
N. ASCUNCE and A. DEL MORAL 47

Breast Cancer Screening in Montpellier
J.-L. LAMARQUE, J. CHERIF CHEIKH, J. PUJOL, P. BOULET, J.-C. LAURENT
and J.-P. DAURES 55

The Bas-Rhin Model: A Non-Centralised Screening Programme
B. GAIRARD, R. RENAUD, P. SCHAFFER and C. GULDENFELS 59

Non-Invasive Breast Cancer: An Important Screening Problem
I. ANDERSSON and D. M. IKEDA 65

Criteria for Recall and Diagnostic Assessment
S. CIATTO and M. ROSSELLI DEL TURCO 79

Pathology in Breast Cancer Screening: A 15-Year Experience from a
Swedish Programme
A. GAD 87

Therapeutic Aspects of Screen-Detected Lesions: The Role of the Surgeon
R. BLAMEY 103

Monitoring the Impact of a Breast Cancer Screening Programme
E. Paci and N. E. Day 111

Training in Mammographic Screening
E. J. Roebuck and A. R. M. Wilson 121

Quality Control in Mammography
A. E. Kirkpatrick 131

Quality of Life and Breast Cancer Screening
J. C. J. M. de Haes and H. J. de Koning 143

Introduction

Adel Gad [1] and Marco Rosselli Del Turco [2]

1   Department of Pathology and Cytology, Falun Hospital, 79 182 Falun, Sweden
2   Centro per lo Studio e la Prevenzione Oncologica, Viale A. Volta 171, 50131 Florence, Italy

In the early 1980s, approximately 250,000 women were enrolled in mammographic screening programmes for early detection of breast cancer, either in controlled studies (Two Counties, Sweden) or in demonstration projects (Utrecht/Nijmegen, the Netherlands; Florence, Italy; UK trial, UK).

Results of these studies have led to the implementation of several other screening programmes on a national or regional basis, which are presently inviting approximately 8-9 million women to periodic mammographic examination. An equal, or even greater number of asymptomatic women refer themselves for mammography with preventive purposes, in the absence of an organised screening programme.

The European Group for Breast Cancer Screening, founded in 1982 in Florence, represented a unique opportunity for breast cancer screening pioneers to exchange their experiences and to discuss results and organisational problems. The Group has produced guidelines for the scientific community, which have been adopted in many ongoing programmes, and it has greatly contributed to the development of mammographic screening all over Europe.

Most studies of breast cancer screening and the largest screening programmes have been performed in Europe and the evidence provided by these experiences is of paramount importance for the design of newly implemented programmes all over the world.

Ten years after its foundation, the European Group for Breast Cancer Screening, in cooperation with the European School of Oncology, has produced this monograph, which deals with the most urging questions concerning breast cancer screening. How, when and where should new screening programmes be implemented? What are the standards and the modalities for the quality control of the different phases of the screening process? How should the existing resources be properly allocated to achieve a relevant reduction in breast cancer mortality?

Screening for breast cancer in women over the age of 50 is one of the possible strategies for the fight against cancer, its efficacy has been scientifically demonstrated and it deserves to be implemented on a large scale as a current health policy. Nevertheless, there are still open questions about breast cancer screening, such as the treatment of screen-detected lesions, how to reduce the frequency of interval cancers, and the efficacy of screening before the age of 50. These and many other issues for research should be stimulated as well as the implementation of organised screening.

Each country will decide how much to invest on breast cancer screening according to its resources and priorities, but all existing programmes should be properly monitorised, the same quality control standards should be adopted, and a common database should be implemented to evaluate and compare the outcome of screening.

We believe that the European Group for Breast Cancer Screening should represent a meeting point for all operators involved in breast cancer screening, to compare and discuss the different experiences and to promote research, training and quality control all over Europe.

Breast Cancer: The Scene in Europe

F. de Waard

Department of Epidemiology, University of Utrecht, Radboudkwartier 261, 3511 CK Utrecht, The Netherlands

In their widely cited monograph on screening, Wilson and Jungner [1] have formulated a number of criteria which have to be fulfilled before screening can be justified. The first of them reads that the disease under consideration should pose an important public health problem either by its prevalence, its severity, or both.

In Northern and Western Europe, breast cancer is undoubtedly a public health problem on both grounds. The cumulative incidence rate over a woman's life time (assuming a life expectancy of 80 years) amounts to a 10% risk of disease occurrence.

With a 10-year survival time of about 40%, there is indeed a clear case for action.

In Eastern and Southern Europe, incidence rates are considerably lower. Figure 1 documents the situation in the EC [2]. It would, however, be useful to have more data from the Mediterranean countries.

One wonders why the differences are so great. In a recent study [3], we were able to show that the variation in incidence rates within Europe can to a large extent be explained by the well-known risk factors, i.e., age at first birth and body weight.

If Eastern and Southern Europe will socio-

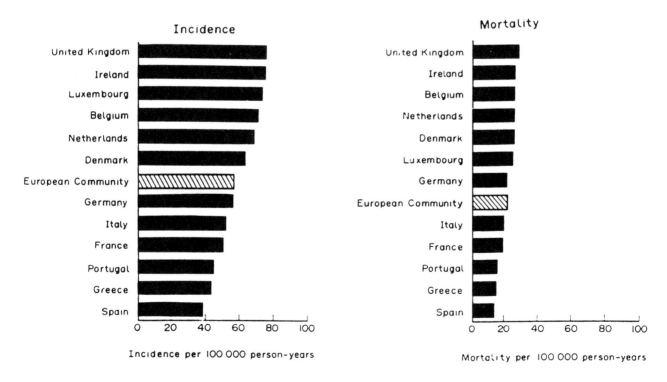

Fig. 1. Estimated incidence and mortality of cancer of the female breast in EC countries [2]

economically catch up in the decade to come with the West and North of Europe, this will probably mean an increase in the incidence of breast cancer. Thus, in the foreseeable future they may also decide that active public health intervention is necessary. Therefore, an interest in mammographic screening is already apparent in the Southern member states of the European Community.

After the publication of the first results of the pioneer study by Strax et al. in New York, screening programmes were developed in Sweden, Italy, the United Kingdom and the Netherlands. These studies have often been discussed and it does not seem necessary to repeat their results here. However, sufficient success has been achieved in women over 50 years of age to convince the health authorities in Sweden, Finland, the United Kingdom and the Netherlands to set up national screening programmes.

In the framework of the EC programme "Europe Against Cancer" launched in 1986, breast screening projects have been developed in Ireland, Belgium, France, Spain, Portugal and Greece, according to common guidelines. Each centre has by now gained experience in screening at least 10,000 women. The centres have learned the art of paying equal attention to high specificity (with a high predictive value of a positive test) and to high sensitivity.

Whereas the designs of the projects and the measures taken to ensure high quality of screening and diagnostic assessment can be harmonised to some extent, the social setting of the various projects remains different. In mountainous regions of Central Portugal, Navarra and the Western Peloponnesos for instance, women have to be brought by minibus to regional centres where mobile units are stationed for some weeks. Even more important than the physical environment are the administrative infrastructure of the regions concerned and the sociocultural context which determine participation rates of the various target populations. Without minimising the efforts and achievement in the other centres, the striking success of the Public Health Department in the Spanish province of Navarra in obtaining 85% participation should be mentioned.

A centralised approach in population screening is apparently not everywhere possible in Europe. This problem relates to health initiatives as well as to the role of vested interests by the medical profession. In Strasbourg, Professor Renaud and co-workers have intelligently sought to overcome the latter problem by persuading all 70 radiologists in the Bas Rhin area to cooperate in a programme of mammographic screening according to common guidelines. All of them send their mammograms to Strasbourg headquarters (called Adémas) for a second reading. Results are fed into a computer enabling the project team to compare results and thereby adding an element of postgraduate education to the programme.

I would not be surprised if this design would be an example to be followed in those regions where a centrally organised programme encounters resistance. Of course, the coordinating centre should build sufficient authority into the design in order to ensure quality control.

One of the targets of the European action against cancer for 1994 is dissemination of screening activities concerning cancers of the breast and cervix uteri. As far as breast cancer is concerned, it would appear justified to stop service programmes for women under the age of 50 since this would put a stop to the ongoing discussion on the merits of mammographic screening.

Within Europe of the Twelve, we look forward to seeing Denmark involved in breast cancer screening; given their infrastructure they should be able to make a success of it. The same holds for Norway and Iceland. Germany and Luxemburg might look to Strasbourg, and perhaps this recipe might also apply to Switzerland and Austria.

It is at present difficult to say whether mammographic breast cancer screening has a high priority in public health action in Eastern European countries. Breast cancer incidence is definitely lower than in North West Europe and it could be that when comparing cost versus effects other choices would be made. It goes without saying that European solidarity nowadays is strong enough to provide our neighbours with advice on how to implement a screening programme as soon as they feel fit for such endeavour.

REFERENCES

1 Wilson JMG, Jungner G: Principles and practice of screening for disease. Public Health Papers nr 34, World Health Organisation, Geneva 1968

2 Moller Jensen O, Esteve J, Moller H, Renard H: Cancer in the European Community and its member states. Eur J Cancer 1990 (27):1167-1256

3 Baanders AN, de Waard F: Breast cancer in Europe; the importance of factors operating at an early age. Eur J Cancer Prevention 1992 (1):285-291

Overview of European Screening Programmes

Leo Pas [1] and Bernt-Peter Robra [2]

1   Cancer Prevention Centre of the Free University of Brussels and Brussels Project on Breast Cancer Screening and Flemish Institute of General Practitioners, De Burburelaan 38, 1970 Wezembeek-Oppem, Belgium
2   Institute of Social Medicine, Epidemiology and Public Health, Magdeburg Medical School, Leipziger Strasse 40, 0-3090 Magdeburg, Germany

Service Screening and Pilot Programmes

Following the series of trials looking into the effectiveness of screening, we are presented with a new challenge: will it be possible to transfer the knowledge thus obtained to a wider population and, thereby, produce similar results within the everyday setting to those carried out within a strongly motivated trial scenario? Will it be possible to keep a firm check on quality and costs?

On the basis of increasing evidence in favour of mammographic breast cancer screening, the United Kingdom, the Netherlands and Sweden are implementing nationwide screening programmes for breast cancer. The Danish Board of Health also recommended the Danish counties to set up breast cancer screening, but only one county (Copenhagen) has begun such a programme.

A number of local programmes are running in other parts of Europe, encouraged, largely, by the European Community: the "Europe Against Cancer" programme co-sponsors a number of pilot projects in Belgium (Brussels and Flanders), France (Strasbourg), Greece (Athens), Ireland (Dublin), Spain (Navarra) and Portugal (Coimbra). The projects are co-coordinated and training facilities are centralised.

It is important, in countries with less experience in mammographic screening, to organise pilot projects before setting up screening programmes on a larger scale. The objective of a pilot project is to define future policy, which can be of 2 kinds: feasibility studies, which will plan at a local level the manpower, resources and organisation modalities required for further programmes, and comparative studies on the diverse organisational modalities (medical, psycho-social and financial aspects).

That there should be a need for **organised** screening programmes has been amply demonstrated by an analysis of cervical cancer screening. Reductions in mortality in the overall population were observed especially wheresoever there was an organised approach, as opposed to those areas where no such programme was installed. Such "opportunistic screening" tends to reach the groups of a lower age and at a lower risk.

We will therefore consider only those programmes with a clearly defined target population, clearly defined procedures to reach this population and elementary monitoring and with at least 10,000 recruited women.

Programme Differences

In countries with free access to mammography, a considerable increase in equipment and mammography performance outside official programmes has been observed (France, Belgium). In Belgium, for instance, a two-fold increase in mammographic activity can be identified from health-insurance data over the past 3 years.

The general characteristics of the different European programmes are similar, but divergences are related to historical background or local characteristics of health services, territory or cultures.

Examples

In the **United Kingdom**, a governmental Committee, chaired by Sir Patrick Forest, recommended the establishment of fixed regional screening centres. Women in the 50-64 age group are invited from the lists of family practitioners, whereas women over 65 will not be invited but can be screened on request. The routine interval has been fixed at 3 years.

The British screening programme has been preceded by a national trial based in 4 centres (Guildford, Edinburgh, Nottingham and Huddersfield). Together with Manchester, 3 of them became the official reference and training centres for the programme.

The Primary Health Care teams of the National Health Service provide correct addresses to the family health authority services, excluding non-eligible women by checking "prior notification lists" sent to them by the inviting office, examine the motivation of women to respond to the invitation and refer for further assessment. Social and emotional aspects can be dealt with either at the screening centre or at the primary health-care level.

Health services in **Italy** are regionalised. The regions differ in their stage of service development. The availability of diagnostic mammography differs along a north-south gradient. Based on the detailed evaluation of a screening centre and a local cancer registry set up in 1970, a pace-setting programme was started in Florence.

The cancer screening programme of the statutory health-insurance system in **Germany** includes a physical examination of the breast and instructions for breast self examination for all women aged 30 and over. Mammography is foreseen for high-risk women (positive family history or previous abnormalities) and for diagnostic purposes. Approximately 1,700 units examine 2.5 million women each year. Hence mammography is already freely available. Screening mammography for symptomless women is not included yet in the health-insurance package. In the former German Democratic Republic, about 100 mammographic units are available but most of them will have to be replaced for technical reasons. The German Mammography Study has been assigned to develop training and quality assurance in preparation for mammographic screening. Two service regions of 34 mammographic units (41 physicians) are involved. Women of 40 years and older are invited by post. The first 3 invitations take place on an annual basis, after which a 2-yearly interval will be recommended.

Screening Modalities (see Table 1)

Age Range

Although the efficacy of mammographic screening on the reduction of mortality in women under the age of 50 has not been proved, some programmes start at a lower age. The Swedish Board of Health is re-examining data with a view to including younger women. In the United Kingdom, a trial comprising 160,000 women in the 40-49 age group has been activated in order to determine the efficacy of mammography in this age group. Assuming a mortality reduction of 8%, models drawn up on data from the Dutch pilot areas show that increasing coverage in the older age-groups is certainly more cost-effective.

Interval

According to the prevailing knowledge that 2-3 yearly intervals are sufficient to obtain the mortality reduction aimed at, intervals of 2 years are most common. In the United Kingdom, the national programme started with a 3-yearly interval. A trial on different screening intervals is now running in the United Kingdom. In Sweden younger women are submitted to an interval of 18 months.

Number of Views

At the initial screen, common consensus is that a 2-view mammogram will effect a de-

Table 1. European mammography programmes (> 10,000 women)

Territory covered	Pilot Service	Start MX	Invited	Age range	MI	PE	Mobile/fixed units
Belgium							
Brussels	P	1992	110,000	50-69	2/1	+/-	F d
Ghent	P	1992	15,000	40-64	2/1	+/-	F d
Flanders	P	1989	45,000	50-64	1	+/-	M
Denmark							
Copenhagen	P	1989	150,000	50-69	2/1		F
Finland	S	1987	275,000	50-62			Fc/d
France							
Strasbourg	P	1989	73,000	50-64	1	+	F d
Rhone	P	1987		50-69	1		F d
Arcades	P	1989	80,000	50-65	1		F d
Sarthe	P	1989	60,000	50-69	1		F d
Montpellier	P	1990		40-70	2		M
Germany							
National Mammography	S	1971		30+	High risk	+	F d
Study	P	1989	600,000	40+	2	+	F d
Greece							
Ilia	P	1989	21,500	40-65	2	-	M
Iceland	S	1989	250,000	40-69	2		SM
Ireland							
Dublin	P	1989	35,000	50-64	2		
Italy							
Florence	P	1970	35,000	40-70*	2	-	M
	S	1990	64,000	50-70	2	-	F/M
Torino	P	1991	144,000	50-69	1	-	F d
Brescia		1987	25,000	50-60	2	+	
Cossata		1989	17,000	50-70			
Massa		1989	15,500	40-70			
Val Trompia		1988	12,611	50-70			
Luxembourg	S	1992	34,000	50-65	2		F d
Netherlands	S	1990	1,500,000	50-69	2/1	-	mix
Portugal							
Coimbra	P	1990	140,000	45-55	1		M
Spain							
Navarra	S	1991	60,000	45-65	1	-	mix
Sweden	S	1989		40-54	2/1	-	F/mix
				55-74	1		
United Kingdom	S	1990	4,000,000	50-64	1	-	mix

PE = physical examination; F = fixed units; c = centralised units; d = decentralised units; M = mobile units; SM = semi-mobile units; mix = combination of mobile and fixed units; + = yes; - = no
* Since 1990, the lower age limit shifted to 50; the "new 40s" will thus not be invited.

crease in the number of women recalled thanks to the increased positive predictive value of mammographic interpretation. The financial benefit from 1 view would be counterbalanced by many technical recalls. Two views are performed in most programmes, but will be followed more often by 1 view in subsequent rounds (except in dense breasts) (2/1). For the same reason, some health authorities in the United Kingdom (45%) offer 2-view mammography at the first round, departing from the national minimal requirements.

Centralised Mammography Services

Except for the HIP study, the original pilot studies and trials all operated in centralised health-service systems in which 1 centre could address women from a large population.

Extension of screening centres to decentralised systems with more liberal access to services, based on fee-for-service, is not likely to be accepted by the medical profession. In such a situation, involvement of private radiologists in centrally coordinated screening programmes would be tested.

A centralised mammographic service can be defined as the provision of 1 screening unit to a defined population (c in Table 1). In a decentralised approach, a high number of mammographic units will serve the population (d in Table 1). Such an organisation prevails in mid-European countries with a fee-for-service payment and a high proportion of privately functioning radiologists (Belgium, France, Luxemburg and Germany).

In Finland, one third of practising radiologists (approximately 100) are working on a part-time basis in screening centres run and co-financed by the cancer society and the municipal health service; some are run in a special municipality-owned health examination company. All radiologists have been specifically trained.

Mobility of Screening Units

In Iceland, women are regularly taken to central units for cervical screening. Semi-mobile units for mammographic screening are transported to such places at appropriate intervals for the target population.

The more dispersed populations in remote areas (Wales, Scotland, Cornwall in the United Kingdom; non-coastal area in Portugal) can be reached by mobile units.

Such mobile units are generally connected to more centrally placed fixed units (F in Table 1).

In mixed systems, the central units generally send the invitations, coordinate the programme, perform film reading and further assessment. Daylight processing may be performed in mobile units, allowing the positioning and quality of the image to be checked on the spot. Mammograms are generally read at the central office from where the invitations are sent.

In the Greek pilot project a mobile unit serves the area, but women are still brought from remote rural areas to the mobile unit.

Access

In countries where the medical profession is paid on a fee-for-service basis (Belgium, Germany, France, Luxemburg), the role of primary care physicians and gynaecologists is fundamental in encouraging women to undergo a mammography. Physical examination may or may not be performed by these physicians (+/-). If physical examination is performed, the population sent to mammographic screening will be asymptomatic, while symptomatic women are referred directly to diagnostic assessment (Strasbourg, Brussels, Germany). The extent to which self-referred women will participate may also largely vary: in Strasbourg, women have direct access to the involved units, while in Brussels the women must first see a physician, although they may be directly transferred.

In the United Kingdom acceptance of self-referred women will depend on the local policy of the health authority.

Assessment

The place where assessment is performed differs according to the national health-service structure and can be either performed in a setting linked to the screening clinic or in the habitual hospital health-service setting.

The Swedish, Italian, Dutch and British assessment systems are described in the chapter by Dr. B. Thomas in this monograph.

In the Belgian, French, Luxembourg and German programmes, assessment can be performed both in the hospital sector and in the outpatient sector. In these countries, consensus and training meetings must stimulate adequate approaches.

Systematic Population Approach

The effectiveness of screening largely depends on the population coverage. Systematic invitation by letter is considered a very efficacious way of recruiting women to screening centres. Such invitations should be centrally issued and be based on an accurate population registry.

In the United Kingdom, the family health authority services provide addresses based on general practitioners' lists, which may pose problems of accuracy, although recent computerisation should have solved some of these problems.

In the Scandinavian countries, the unique personal identification number largely facilitates invitation and monitoring of screening based on accurate population registries.

In the Netherlands, the use of population registries depend on the cooperation of municipalities. Accuracy of the database is good, but sometimes local authorities set other priorities.

The pilot project in Strasbourg does not operate systematic invitations as the electoral lists are not satisfactory, but an extensive population information campaign has been set up, prepared by a population survey. Women are expected to be referred through their family physician or gynaecologist.

The French project in Montpellier has introduced interpersonal mobilisation of women by voluntary groups of women in addition to systematic invitation based on electoral lists. Such programmes might result in a high rate of self-referred women. As this may influence the results selectively, the effects of such organisations must be carefully assessed before they can be extended widely.

In Germany, a multiphase screening programme has existed on a national level since 1971. It is based on the annual sending of an "authorisation form" to the people.

The national Luxembourg programme will operate in the same way.

In highly mobile populations, populations with lower socio-economic level or of different ethnic groups, problems may arise with written invitations. Such problems have been identified for instance in inner cities (London, Manchester). In such cases, systematic invitation may be insufficient and opportunistic, and self-referred women or special campaigns may be needed.

Quality Assurance Systems

The previous screening trials have set the standards for quality assurance, with daily recording of baseline parameters for processing performance, maintenance prescriptions, and regular image quality control.

In the Netherlands, all screening units are linked by modem to a central reference unit in Nijmegen. Daily running parameters are checked against a standard and authorisation is given to start the mammography.

Originally, double reading was not required in the highly motivated and experienced trial centres. With the extension of screening to service level, the reference centres performed *de facto* double reading due to continuous availability of trainees. Pilot projects sponsored by the European community all involve double reading of mammograms as a rule.

In the Strasbourg pilot project, double reading is one of the major features of the quality-assurance programme. It allows for monitoring image quality in a decentralised system by private radiologists. This provides private radiologists with an opportunity for coordination and training in a liberally functioning health-service system. This process is likely to increase sensitivity and specificity in such a situation.

Monitoring Systems

The monitoring of programmes should essentially be based on the linkage of individual data concerning invitation, participation, the results of screening tests and further work-up procedures. In the case of positivity, invitation and participation lists, screening results and follow-up data must be gathered in a central computerised database. Moreover, interval cancer can be identified through cancer registries, thereby defining the sensitivity of the programme.

If such registries are absent, it is recommended that they be created together with the planning of projects or service screening. They particularly allow early parameters of efficacy to be determined and proper action to be taken in the case of observed deficiencies. In the Netherlands, a special monitoring system has been set up in collaboration with the Regional Cancer Control Offices. Data are merged in an automated central database for epidemiologic monitoring. Coding and access are strictly regulated.

Planning

Given the multidisciplinary functions of breast cancer screening and its extension to service level, particular attention should be given to formal coordination.

The screening units in Sweden are generally linked to a hospital in a centralised health system. Screening, assessment and treatment decisions are regularly discussed in multidisciplinary meetings involving screening staff, cytologists, pathologists and surgeons.

In the United Kingdom, coordinators appointed locally are responsible for the good functioning of the programmes, with particular emphasis on participation, quality assurance and follow-up of screen-detected lesions. National coordinating groups have been set up dealing with the programme coordination of different aspects such as quality assurance, pathology reporting and proficiency testing, and primary health-care coordination.

In the Strasbourg pilot centre, a formal contract is signed with private radiologists to assure their adherence to the principles of the programme. In return, the insurance system reimburses them with a special fee for screening.

The Brussels project has formally involved physicians from all professions in a local society to evolve the detailed practical modalities of the programme and set standards of care.

Conclusion

The technical basis of mammographic screening is identical but the way service programmes can be conceived largely depends on local health-service characteristics and available resources, of which adequate manpower is an essential part.

Programmes differ largely in the way the target population is recruited, the number of units required for this population, the way the link with the curative health sector is structured, and the facilities available for monitoring.

Such modalities will define the effectiveness and the costs. The varied experience of pioneers and pilot project members of the European Group for Breast Cancer Screening will ensure further refinement of our knowledge in adapting the technique to local settings.

FURTHER READING

1   Austoker J: Breast cancer screening and primary care team. Br Med J 1990 (300):1631-1634

2   Committee of Cancer Experts: Recommendations on breast cancer screening. European Community, Brussels 1992

3   Cruz DB, Alves JC, Rodrigues VL: Screening of cancer of the breast in central Portugal. Pathol Biol Paris 1992 (39):848-849

4   European Group for Breast Cancer Screening: Recommendations for breast cancer screening. Eur J Gynaecol Oncol 1990 (11:6):489-490

5   Forrest AP: Breast cancer: the decision to screen. J Public Health Med 1991 (13:1):2-12

6   Gad A, Thomas BA, Moskowitz M: Screening for breast cancer in Europe: achievements, problems and future. Recent results. Cancer Res 1984 (90):180-194

7   Hislop GT, Warren BJ, Basco VE, Vincent TY, Math M: The screening mammography program of British Columbia: pilot study. Cancer J Public Health 1991 (82):168-173

8   Hogod C, Fog J: Screening: why, when and how? National Board of Health, Denmark 1992

9   Hurley SF, Jolly DJ, Livingston PM, Reading D, Cocurn J, Flint Richeter D: Effectiveness, costs and cost-effectiveness of recruitment strategies for a mammographic screening program to detect breast cancer. JNCI 1992 (84:11):863-865

10 Lamarque JL, Pujol H, Daures JP et al: The Montpellier experience. Pathol Biol Paris 1992 (39:9):852

11 Pamilo M, Antinen I, Soiva M, Roiha M, Suramo I: Mammographic screening - reasons for recall and the influence of experience on recall in the Finnish system. Clin Radiol 1990 (41):384-387

12 Pas L: Outlines for Cancer Prevention Through Primary Health Care. Vlaams Huisartsen Instituut, Antwerp 1992

13 Renaud R: Basic principles of breast cancer screening. J Gynaecol Obstet Biol Reprod 1987 (16):565-577

14 Renaud R, Schaffer P, Gairard B, Dale G, Haehnel P, Kleitz C, Guldenfels C: Principles and first results of the European screening campaign for breast cancer in the Bas-Rhin. Bull Acad Natle Méd 1991 (175):129-147

15 Rosselli Del Turco M: Breast cancer screening programme: the Italian experience. Pathol Biol Paris 1992 (39:9):850-851

Evidence of the Effectiveness of Breast Cancer Screening

Jocelyn Chamberlain [1] and Domenico Palli [2]

1 The Institute of Cancer Research, Royal Cancer Hospital, D H Cancer Screening Evaluation Unit, 15 Cotswold Road, Sutton, Surrey SM2 5NG, United Kingdom
2 Centro per lo Studio e la Prevenzione Oncologica, Epidemiology Unit, Viale A. Volta 171, 50131 Florence, Italy

Because screening is offered by the medical profession to supposedly well women in the general public, there is a particular ethical responsibility to be certain that it is effective in its implicit purpose of saving lives, and that the level of benefit it offers outweighs its costs and disadvantages to the women concerned. A large amount of research has therefore been undertaken to measure the value of screening for breast cancer.

Soon after setting up a screening programme, there are 3 measures that are commonly claimed to indicate that it is beneficial, namely (i) a yield of cancer greater than the expected incidence, (ii) a shift to an earlier stage distribution, and (iii) a lower case-fatality rate among screen-detected cases than among symptomatic cancers. These findings are common to all breast cancer screening programmes but, while they are necessary concomitants of successful screening, on their own they are insufficient to prove that deaths from breast cancer are being prevented. It could be that screening is merely advancing the date of diagnosis of tumours of low malignant potential that would not prove lethal, even if left until they were symptomatic. It is perhaps worth pointing out why case-fatality rates are not so useful in evaluating screening as they are in evaluating the effects of different treatments. There are several factors, each of which biases case-fatality comparisons in favour of screen-detected cases. Firstly, case-fatality rates are expressed in terms of the proportion of cases which have died within a set time from diagnosis. Screening advances the date of diagnosis and therefore automatically extends the period between diagnosis and death; this is known as *lead-time bias*. Secondly, the type of women who take up the offer of screening are likely to be health-aware women who would, even in the absence of screening, present early with symptoms and have a good prognosis. This is called *selection bias* and is well illustrated by the fact that in most of the prospective trials discussed below, women who did not attend for screening had a higher breast cancer mortality rate than women in the control group. Thirdly, slowly growing tumours spend a longer time than aggressive fast growing tumours in the phase when they are pre-symptomatic but detectable by screening; therefore, the cases detected by screening contain an excess proportion of slowly growing cancers and a deficit of cancers with high malignant potential and this *length bias* clearly affects case-fatality comparisons. Finally, an extreme form of length bias is the detection by screening of apparently malignant lesions which, had they not been screened, would have remained latent and undiagnosed throughout the woman's life-time. This *over-diagnosis bias* is likely to apply particularly to cases diagnosed at the prevalent screen and possibly also to cases detected in the *in-situ* phase. All these biases make case-fatality comparisons inappropriate for evaluation of screening.

If case-fatality rates are inadequate, which alternatives are available? The answer is to compare the number of breast cancer deaths in a whole population for whom screening has been provided and a population for whom it has not, in other words, using breast cancer deaths per women in the population as the indicator rather than breast cancer deaths per patient.

There are a number of different epidemiological study designs which can be employed to compare breast cancer mortality rates among populations with and without screening programmes. The methods and their main findings are described below.

Prospective Randomised Controlled Trials

This ideal study design involves identifying a population of women (none of whom have diagnosed breast cancer at entry to the trial) and randomly allocating them either to a study group who are offered screening or to a control group who are not. All breast cancers diagnosed in both groups over the ensuing years are recorded; it should be noted that in the study group the breast cancers are not only those detected by screening but include also cancers presenting symptomatically at an interval after a negative screen (interval cases), and cancers presenting among women who did not attend. This is because these non-screen-detected cancers must have their counterparts in the control group. Eventually a comparison is made between the number of deaths from breast cancer in the total study and control groups.

The Health Insurance Plan (HIP) of Greater New York Trial

This classic study was started in New York in 1963 [1]. Its design and main findings are illustrated in Figure 1. Sixty-two thousand women aged 40 to 64 who were members of the Health Insurance Plan were randomly allocated to study or control groups. Those in the study group were individually invited to be screened by mammography and physical examination of the breasts on 4 occasions at annual intervals. Screening then stopped. The mortality comparison is restricted to breast cancer deaths among women whose cancer was diagnosed during the first 5 years because by this time the number of breast cancers in the control group had caught up with the number in the study group, indicating a comparable case-mix in both groups. A

mortality difference in favour of the study group began to appear within about 4 years of entry and reached its maximum between 5 and 7 years, then being maintained for the remainder of the 18 year follow-up. The mortality reduction was 38% at 5 years, 29% at 10 years and 23% at 18 years.

The Swedish Two-County Trial

Following the early promising results from the HIP study [2], a number of other investigations were set up to confirm or refute the benefit of screening. The first of these was the Swedish Two-County study [3] in which 133,065 women aged 40 to 74 and resident in Kopparberg and Ostergötland Counties were randomised into study and control groups, the units of randomisation being parishes, not individuals. In Kopparberg, 2 parishes were allocated to the study group for every one allocated to the control group, and in Ostergötland they were evenly split, resulting in 77,080 women in the study group and 55,985 controls. Women in the study group were invited for screening by single oblique view mammography and almost 90% accepted. The average interval between screens was 22 months for women aged 40 to 49, and 33 months for women aged 50 to 74. After an average follow-up of 7.9 years, there was a 31% reduction in breast cancer mortality in the study group significant at the 0.001 level.

The Malmö Trial

The next trial to report its findings was another randomised controlled trial from Sweden, in the city of Malmö [4]. Women aged 45 to 70 were individually randomised to study (21,088) or control group (21,195). Seventy-four percent of the study group attended for screening, which was by 2-view mammography, with screening repeated at 18 to 24-month intervals. During the first 7 years of the trial, breast cancer mortality was higher in the study group than the controls but by 10 years, cumulative mortality in the study group was marginally lower (4%). The investigators were extremely careful to verify the cause of death in each breast cancer case,

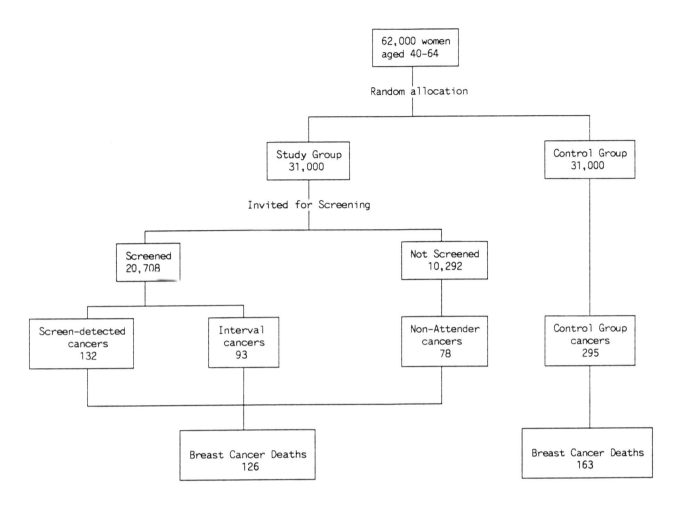

Fig. 1. Summary of HIP study, showing cancers diagnosed within 5 years from entry; and breast cancer deaths among them up to 18 years from entry [1]

but the study had 2 problems, firstly considerable contamination of the control group, 25% of whom had a mammogram, and secondly an insufficient sample size to give the trial statistical power. Thus, there is a wide zone of uncertainty around the point estimate of a 4% mortality reduction (95% CI 32% to -35%). Nevertheless, the findings of such an insignificant effect threw doubt on the optimistic estimates of benefit reported by the first 2 trials.

The Edinburgh Trial

Another randomised trial was started in Edinburgh, Scotland, in 1979 [5]. The units for randomisation were general practices, virtually the whole population being on the list of a general practitioner. Forty-five thousand women aged 45 to 64 were identified on the lists of the general practices in the study, and randomisation resulted in 23,226 in the study group and 21,904 in the control group. Women in the study group were invited for screening by physical examination every year for 7 years, and mammography was also provided at the first, third, fifth and seventh rounds; only 61% of invited women attended for screening. After 7 years mortality was 17% lower in the study group than the control group, but the 95% confidence intervals were wide (42% to 18%) and the difference is not statistically significant.

The Stockholm Trial

In Stockholm, Sweden, 60,000 women aged 40 to 64 were individually randomised into a study group (40,000) or a control group

(20,000). Screening was by single oblique view mammography alone, with an average interval of 28 months between screening rounds, and 82% of study group women were screened at least once. A preliminary analysis with an average follow-up of 7 years showed a 24% reduction which again was not statistically significant [6].

Thus, the 3 most recent trials, although consistent with the conclusion that screening saves lives, gave less optimistic estimates of the level of benefit that could be achieved and none were statistically significant. One important point is that none had a large enough sample size to give the trial sufficient statistical power to prove or reject the hypothesis. The power of a trial is crucially dependent on the number of deaths in the control group as well as on the level of mortality reduction it is intended to prove or disprove, and none of these trials seem to have calculated in advance the expected deaths in a control cohort of women free from diagnosed breast cancer at entry [7].

Prospective Geographical Comparisons

A study design similar to that of a randomised controlled trial is used in comparing breast cancer mortality in geographical areas with different screening provision, although because the women are not randomly allocated there may be underlying factors, other than the screening intervention, contributing to a mortality difference, and more cautious interpretation is required.

The UK Trial of Early Detection of Breast Cancer

Between 1979 and 1981 this trial enrolled nearly 240,000 women aged 45 to 64 living in 8 geographically separate districts in the United Kingdom [8]. Two districts invited 45,956 women to be screened annually for 7 years by physical examination with mammography in alternate rounds (the study group of the Edinburgh trial mentioned above was one

of these districts). Two more districts invited 63,571 women to a teaching session to learn about breast self-examination (BSE) and also provided a diagnostic breast clinic which women could freely use. The remaining 4 districts, in which 127,109 women were identified but not contacted, served as a control group. As well as keeping a record of screening and BSE class attendance, all breast histology (benign as well as malignant) in these women in all 8 districts was recorded, together with deaths from breast cancer and from all causes. Acceptance of screening was 67%, but only 45% of women accepted the invitation to a BSE class; a sample interview survey found that one year later 41% of women in one of the BSE districts were performing BSE adequately compared with 27% in one of the control districts (p < 0.01) [9].

After 10 years of follow-up, there was a statistically significant 20% reduction in breast cancer mortality in the combined screening districts compared with the combined comparison districts, although the 95% confidence intervals are still wide, consistent with anything from a 5% to a 33% reduction. There was no difference in mortality between the BSE districts combined and the comparison districts.

The Utrecht Study

In the Netherlands, the city of Utrecht started a screening programme in 1974 for women aged 50 to 64 (and subsequently for younger cohorts) [10]. All women aged 50 to 64 were invited for screening by physical examination and mammography on 5 occasions at increasing intervals, and 72% were screened at least once. A comparison between Utrecht and 17 other Dutch cities with no screening showed that breast cancer mortality among women born between 1911 and 1925 rose steadily over the 13-year period from 1970 to 1983 in the other cities but in Utrecht it levelled off in the late 1970s, resulting in an increasing gap between Utrecht and the others. While it is not possible to put a quantitative estimate on the mortality reduction this represents, the pattern is similar to that seen in the more formal trials.

Conclusions from Prospective Trials

All of the studies described above address the public health question of how many breast cancer deaths can be avoided by a population-based screening programme. A statistical meta-analysis of the different randomised trials has not been done although an overview of the Swedish trials is currently in progress. Day, combining the trials "naively", suggests that a pooled estimate of the mortality reduction achieved by screening populations of women aged over 50 is 29% (95% confidence intervals 17% to 39%) [11].

As already seen, these population-based controlled trials of necessity include breast cancer deaths among never-screened women in the study group and, depending on the level of compliance, underestimate the percentage mortality reduction among women who actually were screened. Making allowances for compliance and for the fact that mortality in never-attenders exceeded that of the control group in all but the HIP trial, Day gives a conservative estimate of 39% lower mortality among screened women aged over 50. The question of differential effectiveness in different age groups is discussed lated in this chapter.

The failure of the UK trial to show any reduction in mortality in the BSE districts could in part be attributable to low compliance with BSE in comparison with screening compliance. The lack of any demonstrable effect shows that the programme of education was ineffective at the population level, but does not necessarily mean that for individual women breast self-examination is ineffective. This remains an open question.

Retrospective Case-Control Studies

A case-control study design has been used to evaluate screening programmes where no control population was available. Because of the retrospective design, these studies are easier to conduct and have the advantage of low cost. However, problems in the definition of cases and controls and potential sources of biases have been identified and discussed in detail [12,13]. Briefly, cases are women dead from breast cancer diagnosed after the start of the programme, while age-matched controls are randomly sampled from the general population. Their screening histories are recorded up to the date of diagnosis of each case and then compared. The resulting odds ratio is an estimate of the risk of dying from breast cancer of women who accepted to be screened in comparison to women who refused to be screened. While other potential confounding factors can be controlled in the design, the role of selection bias cannot be completely excluded.

In order to compare estimates of mortality reduction provided by case-control studies with those from randomised trials, the compliance of the invited population has to be taken into account. Overall, the agreement is reasonable and results of the case-control studies, carried out in populations with widely different health-care systems and cultural backgrounds, can be considered as supporting the evidence of the mortality reduction shown by randomised trials.

The Dutch Studies

Two case-control studies of breast cancer screening were first published from Nijmegen [14] and Utrecht [10] in The Netherlands. Different results were reported, possibly because of differences in age ranges for invitation (35+ vs 50-64), in other details of study design (case definition) and also in the original screening protocol. The 2 programmes had been started in 1975 and 1974, inviting about 30,000 and 20,000 women, respectively. The Nijmegen study identified 46 cases and found a relative risk of dying from breast cancer of 0.48 (95% CI 0.23-1.00) for screened vs unscreened women; in Utrecht, again 46 cases were studied and the relative risk estimate was even more favourable, namely 0.30 (95% CI 0.13-0.70).

The Florence Study

This programme was started in the Florence district in 1970 but additional towns were involved over the period 1970-81. Overall, at the 1981 census, the female population in the

40-70 age group periodically invited to screening reached 33,000. A first study [15] considering 57 cases dead in the period 1977-84, found a relative risk of 0.53 (95% CI 0.29-0.95) after adjustment for potential confounders (marital status, use of health services and education). This finding was confirmed in an updated analysis 3 years later [16].

Effectiveness in Different Age Groups

One consistent but disappointing finding in all research into the outcome of breast screening is that it is less effective in women aged under 50 when first invited to be screened, and indeed no trial has yet shown a statistically significant difference in this age group. Three trials suggest some benefit, namely the HIP study (25% mortality reduction after 18 years), the Swedish Two-County trial (8% mortality reduction after 9 years) and the UK Trial of Early Detection of Breast Cancer (26% reduction after 10 years). But others suggest an excess mortality in this age group, Malmö finding 29% excess mortality in women aged

less than 55, and Stockholm 7% excess in women below 50. The Edinburgh trial showed virtually no effect in women aged 45 to 49.

All these analyses suffer from lack of statistical power, having very wide confidence intervals surrounding the point estimates of mortality difference. This is illustrated in Figure 2 which shows for each trial the risk of breast cancer death in the study group relative to the control group. Any point less than 1.0 indicates a mortality reduction, more than 1.0 a mortality excess. The bars extending from the point estimates represent 95% confidence intervals, all of which overlap 1.0, the point of no effect.

Similarly in the case-control studies, the highest protection was shown by the Utrecht study [10] in which only women aged 50-64 were invited. In Florence [16] the analysis in the 40-49 age group showed a weaker effect, far from statistical significance, in comparison to older women, but only 28 cases were available. Lack of statistical power in age-group analysis is common, however, but pooling of published case-control studies has not yet been planned.

Further studies, focussing specifically on younger women, are underway in Canada [17] and in the UK [18]. The UK trial is recruiting a cohort of 195,000 women aged 40-41, randomly allocating them to study or control groups and offering the study group annual mammographic screening (2 views) for 7 years. The large sample size will give the trial 80% power to detect a statistically significant 22% mortality reduction (or greater) after 10 years of follow-up.

Thus, on present evidence the benefit of screening women under the age of 50 is uncertain, but it seems likely that with screening as practised in the past, any benefit in terms of mortality reduction is likely to be considerably less than that in older women.

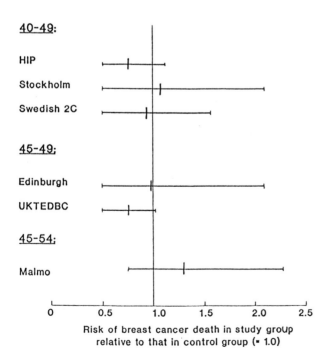

Fig. 2. Summary of results from breast cancer screening trials in women aged 40-54

Sensitivity and Frequency of Screening

One reason contributing to the disappointing findings in younger women is that both mammography and physical examination have poorer sensitivity for cancer detection in pre-menopausal breasts. This is well illustrated in the Swedish Two-County study using the proportional incidence method for estimating sensitivity [19].

The proportional incidence method depends upon knowledge of the expected incidence of breast cancer in screened women if they had not been screened; this can be derived from the control group (after adjusting for incidence in non-responders). Interval cancers occurrring within successive years from negative screening are then subtracted from the number expected if there had been no screening. The remaining number represents those cancers which would have presented that year had they not been detected earlier by screening. This is expressed as a proportion of the expected incidence and represents the sensitivity of the screening test.

Among women aged over 50 in the Swedish Two-County study, in the first 12 months after a negative screen, interval cancers represented 13% of the expected incidence, giving a sensitivity of 87% in the first year. Between 12 and 24 months after a negative screen, interval cancers represented 29% of the expected incidence, giving a sensitivity of 71% in the second year after screening. But in women aged 40-49 there were proportionally more interval cancers and sensitivity was only 62% in the first year after a screen, falling to 32% in the second year. Thus, the ability of screening to detect cancers is clearly much worse in younger women than in those aged 50 or over.

This method of estimating sensitivity in successive time periods after screening clearly also gives useful information for decisions about the frequency with which screening needs to be repeated. Among women over 50, sensitivity in the Two-County trial was shown to fall from 87% in the first year after screening to 71% in the second year, to 55% in the third year. Similarly in Utrecht, which experimented with different intervals, interval cancers rose, approaching the pre-study incidence rate during the fourth year after a negative screen [20].

Most breast screening programmes have opted for an interval of 2 years between routine re-screens, although the UK programme was set up with a 3-year interval, on the basis that in women aged 50 and over a mortality reduction of 40% was seen in the Two-County trial with screening by single-view mammography repeated at an interval of 33 months.

Future Resarch into the Effectiveness of Screening

Many of the unresolved issues regarding policy decisions on provision of screening relate to economic studies of the marginal costs and benefits of alternative strategies, for example by shortening the interval or increasing the number of mammographic views, or using film readers with different qualifications. While it would in theory be desirable to conduct trials to find out the extra lives saved by different strategies and the extra cost per life-years, in practice the vast sample sizes required to measure these marginal benefits and costs mean that proxy endpoints need to be used, with extrapolation by statistical models to estimate changes in life-years.

Within Europe, probably the most pressing question is the value of screening women aged under 50. As already seen, this is currently under investigation but the size and duration of trial required mean that it will be at least a further decade before a reasonably definitive answer to this question will be obtained.

Bearing in mind the rapidly increasing incidence of breast cancer in the developing world, the value of screening by less expensive methods than mammography is a high priority. The International Agency for Research on Cancer is investigating the feasibility of a trial in the Philippines to measure the effectiveness of physical examination in reducing mortality, and a similar trial is being planned in South America. A current study in Canada is looking into the relative effectiveness of physical examination and mammography but as this trial does not have an unscreened control arm, the effect of physical examination alone cannot be obtained from it. Breast self-examination, like other preventive interventions which depend upon health education, is notoriously difficult to evaluate. The negative effect of the BSE education programme in the UK trial should not be taken as conclusive evidence that BSE is ineffective, and further trials are required. One such trial is ongoing in Russia.

Speculating into the future, no doubt new tests suitable for screening will be devised, both in the field of imaging and of biological markers, and these too will need to be evaluated for their effect on benefits and costs. Identification of genetic markers for breast cancer may lead to much more specific definition of risk, thus enabling screening to be focussed only on a small group of high-risk women.

Meanwhile, developments in other means of breast cancer control, either by primary prevention [21] or by improvements in therapy [22], need to be monitored, for it is possible - and highly desirable - that *their* effectiveness in reducing breast cancer mortality may make the proportional contribution of screening much less than its current level of 25-30% within a limited age band.

REFERENCES

1   Shapiro S, Venet W, Strax P, Venet L: Periodic screening for breast cancer. In: The Health Insurance Plan Project and Its Sequelae, 1963-1986. John Hopkins University Press, Baltimore & London 1988

2   Shapiro S, Strax P, Venet L: Periodic breast cancer screening in reducing mortality from breast cancer. JAMA 1971 (215):1777-1785

3   Tabar L, Fagerberg G, Duffy SW, Day NE: The Swedish Two-County trial of mammographic screening for breast cancer: recent results and calculation of benefit. J Epidemiol Community Health 1989 (43):107-114

4   Andersson I, Aspegren K, Janzon L et al: Mammographic screening and mortality from breast cancer: the Malmo mammographic screening trial. Br Med J 1988 (297):943-994

5   Roberts MM, Alexander FE, Anderson TJ et al: Edinburgh trial of screening for breast cancer: mortality at seven years. Lancet 1990 (335):241-246

6   Frisell J, Eklund G, Hellstrom L et al: Randomized study of mammography screening - preliminary report on mortality in the Stockholm trial. Breast Cancer Res Treat 1991 (18):49-56

7   Moss SM, Draper GJ, Hardcastle JD, Chamberlain J: Calculation of sample size in trials for early diagnosis of disease. Int J Epidemiol 1987 (16):104-110

8   UK Trial of Early Detection of Breast Cancer. Breast cancer mortality after ten years in the UK Trial of Early Detection of Breast Cancer (submitted)

9   Calnan MW, Chamberlain J, Moss S: Compliance with a class teaching breast self-examination. J Epidemiol Community Health 1983 (37-4):264-270

10 Collette HJA, Day NE, Rombach JJ, de Waard F: Evaluation of screening for breast cancer in a non-randomised study (the DOM Project) by means of a case-control study. Lancet 1984 (i):1224-1225

11 Day NE: Screening for Breast Cancer. Br Med Bull 1991 (47):400-415

12 Sasco AJ, Day NE, Walter SD: case-control studies for the evaluation of screening. J Chron Dis 1986 (39):399-405

13 Moss SM: Case-control studies of screening. Int J Epidemiol 1991 (20):1-6

14 Verbeek ALM, Hendriks JHCL, Holland R, Mravunac M, Sturmans F, Day NE: Reduction of breast cancer mortality through mass screening with modern mammograph: first results of the Nijmegen project, 1975-1981. Lancet 1984 (i):1222-1224

15 Palli D, Rosselli del Turco M, Buiatti E, Carli S, Ciatto S, Toscani L, Maltoni GC: A case-control study of the efficacy of a non-randomized breast cancer screening program in Florence (Italy). Int J Cancer 1986 (38):501-504

16 Palli D, Rosselli del Turco M, Buiatti E, Ciatto S, Crocetti E, Paci F: Time intervals since last test in a breast cancer screening programme: a case-control study in Italy. J Epidemiol Health 1989 (43):241-248

17 Miller AB, Baines CJ, To T, Wall C: The Canadian National Breast Screening Study. In: Cancer Screening. Miller AB, Chamberlain J, Day NE (eds). Hakama M & Prorok PC. Cambridge University Press, 1991 pp 45-55

18 UKCCCR Subcommittee on Breast Screening Research, UKCCCR-sponsored Research on Breast Cancer Screening. J. Public Health Med. In press

19 Tabar L, Fagerberg G, Day NE, Holmberg L: What is the optimum interval between mammography screening examinations? Br J Cancer 1987 (55):547-551

20 de Waard F, Collette HJA, Rombach JJ, Bannders-van Halewijn EA, Honing C: The DOM project for the early detection of breast cancer, Utrecht, The Netherlands. J Chronic Dis 1984 (37-1):1-44

21 Powles TJ, Hardy SE, Ashley GM, et al: A pilot trial to evalute the acute toxicity and feasibility of tamoxifen for prevention of breast cancer. Br J Cancer 1989 (60):126-131

22 Early Breast Cancer Trialists' Collaborative Group. Effects of adjuvant tamoxifen and of cytotoxic therapy on mortality in early breast cancer. N Engl J Med 1988 (319):1681-1692

Cost-Effectiveness Analysis of Breast Cancer Screening

H.J. de Koning, J.D.F. Habbema, B.M. van Ineveld and G.J. van Oortmarssen

Erasmus University Rotterdam, Department of Public Health and Social Medicine, P.O. Box 1738, 3000 DR Rotterdam, The Netherlands

Methodology of Cost-Effectiveness Analysis

The Approach

There are 3 related types of analysis for assessing relationships between costs, risks and health benefits [1,2], the first one being the cost-effectiveness analysis (CE-analysis). In this case, one effect measure is chosen, e.g. life-years gained, and the analysis tries to define the costs of screening and its effects. For costs one should ideally think of social costs as "opportunity costs", i.e., benefits forgone because the resources are not used for other excellent purposes. Social costs may be quite different from financial streams. A second type of analysis is called cost-utility analysis (CUA), which arises when one is not satisfied with expressing the health benefits and risks of screening in only one effect measure. In the cost-utility analysis, several effect measures are weighted in order to obtain one overall measure for the health effects of screening, called the utility. The best known example of a utility is "quality-adjusted life-years" or QALYs. In this case the life-years are weighted by the quality in which these years are spent. Finally, there is the cost-benefit analysis (CBA). In this case the costs and utility from the cost-utility analysis are traded off by fixing a price value for one unit of utility. Most analyses carried out thus far are cost-effectiveness analyses.

When a cost-effectiveness analysis is supplemented with a number of other considerations, such as organisational aspects, impact on health care needs and demands, legal and ethical issues, it may be called a "medical technology assessment". All 3 types rest on the interdisciplinary research of medical researchers, economists and other disciplines.

Roughly 2 types of cost-effectiveness calculations can be distinguished. The first one considers an idealised birth cohort that is followed from birth to death. This analysis gives useful insight and is easy to interpret from an epidemiological point of view. The second approach, the one we follow, is a real-time, real-population approach. In this case a dynamic population is followed over time, including mortality and births. Moreover, the situation concerning the disease is assessed at the start of the screening and future time trends are superimposed on it.

This second type of cost-effectiveness calculation is more complex than the first type (in practice, one usually starts with exploratory cohort calculations, even when real population analysis is the aim) but it has a number of advantages. The results of a real-population analysis are more useful for policy advice. It is also crucial to assess the impact on needs and demands in the health-care systems. Moreover, it is a natural first step towards later evaluation and monitoring. The real-population type cost-effectiveness analysis requires extensive calculations, and we have therefore developed a computer programme called MISCAN (Micro-simulation Screening Analysis). It simulates individual life histories of women according to specified assumptions, including the natural history of cancer and the impact of screening [3,4].

This chapter discusses the lines along which such a cost-effectiveness analysis has been

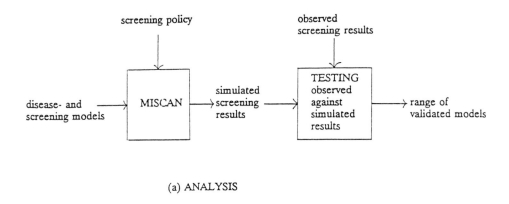

(a) ANALYSIS

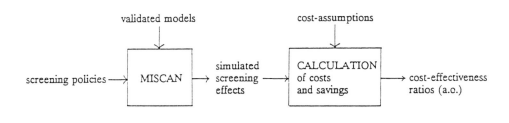

(b) PROSPECTIVE EVALUATION

Fig. 1. The two phases of a cost-effectiveness analysis of screening

carried out. Organisation and decision-making concerning breast cancer screening have been considered in another paper [5]. The main results of the cost-effectiveness analysis have been reported elsewhere [6,7]. The present paper focusses less on results but more on some phases a cost-effectiveness analysis has to go through before it is completed and the types of assumptions to be made during the analysis. If not otherwise indicated, results derive from the 2 reports and the final Dutch report [6-8].

The Analysis Phase

A cost-effectiveness analysis should in the first place be based on the current knowledge of the epidemiology and the natural history of the disease, its preclinical stages and the impact of screening. Therefore, a cost-effectiveness analysis can be broken down into 2 broad phases [9]: a) analysis, in which vali-

dated assumptions on disease process and screening are obtained and b) prospective evaluation, in which the costs, risks and benefits of screening policies are assessed (Fig. 1).

In the analysis phase, the results of screening trials are analysed in order to draw conclusions on the underlying processes concerning disease and screening. In the case of breast cancer screening, use is made of the HIP randomised trial, of the mortality reduction results of the randomised trials in Sweden, and of the studies in Utrecht and Nijmegen in the Netherlands.

The crucial baseline assumption on improvement in prognosis after early (mammographic) detection is based on the reported results from the randomised trials in Kopparberg/Ostergötland [10] and Malmö [11]. Simulating the 2 Swedish programmes separately, and taking into account the specific attendance rate, screening interval, age group and follow-up period for each, the expected effects on breast cancer mortality reduction for both trials were the same. These factors could, therefore, not explain the different published point estimates on mortality reduction. Assuming equal mammographic quality in both projects, we combined the results and calculated a weighted (on trial size) average [7].

Table 1 shows some main results concerning the disease process derived from the analysis. Assumptions are presented concerning the duration of preclinical disease, sensitivity of mammography, and breast cancer mortality reduction.

These assumptions were derived in the analysis phase of the cost-effectiveness study for breast cancer screening. For a description of the analysis phase of MISCAN, see [12].

The Prospective Evaluation Phase

In the evaluation phase, different screening policies have to be assessed for their costs, risks, benefits and other consequences. This requires a large number of other assumptions based on different research. The main ones concern:

Period of Screening
It is assumed that screening will take place during the period 1990-2017 in the Netherlands.

Base-Case
The future developments in case of screening should always be compared with what would happen if there were no screening. We assumed that present age-specific rates of mammographic examination in the Netherlands will also apply during the period 1990-2017.

Situation at Start
We assumed that age-specific incidence, stage-distribution at clinical surfacing and stage-specific survival will remain at the 1988 level during the whole period of screening. We assume population dynamics according to the middle scenario of the Dutch Central Bureau of Statistics.

Screening Policies
The 4 main policies concern screening between the ages of 50 and 70. They differ in the frequency of screening: 5, 10, 15 and 20 screenings during these 20 years. We will especially consider the results of the 10 screenings which, according to the Dutch screening policy, are carried out at ages 51, 53, 55, 57, 59, 61, 63, 65, 67 and 69.

Table 1. Assumptions derived in the analysis phase of the cost-effectiveness study for breast cancer screening

Average duration of the total preclinical screen-detectable stage (age/average duration in years)

40	2.1
50	2.7
60	3.9
70	6.2

Sensitivity of mammography

dCIS	40%
< 10 mm	70%
10-19 mm	95%
≥ 20 mm	95%

Reduction in probability of breast cancer death when breast cancer is detected early (size at detection / reduction in probability)

< 10 mm	64%
10-19 mm	60%
≥ 20 mm	48%

Build-up Phase
It is assumed that during the period 1990-1994 the entire country of the Netherlands will gradually be covered by a network of screening units. The screening units will be fixed, mobile or semi-mobile, depending on the population density in the area.

Costs
Detailed cost studies have been undertaken. From an economic point of view, costs can be divided into direct and indirect costs. Direct costs can again be split up into medical costs and other costs. Costs of different diagnostic and therapeutic procedures and costs of treatment of advanced breast cancer are also assessed as part of the direct medical costs [13,14]. The direct non-medical costs, as well as the indirect costs, have been included in the sensitivity analyses. In this way the contribution to the final results can be clearly distinguished. Indirect costs have as components production losses and medical costs during life-years gained. As the women involved are at least 50 years old, the production losses that will occur are limited. Therefore, this aspect has not been considered within the sensitivity analyses.

Discount Rate
In accordance with recommendations, including those of the Dutch government, a yearly discount rate of 5% has been applied to both costs and effects [15].

Attendance Rate
In accordance with what has been observed in the studies in the Netherlands, attendance rate is assumed to be 75% for women under 50, slowly decreasing to 65% at age 70 and steeply decreasing over 70, to 45% at age 75. Attendance rates differ widely between women who did or did not attend the previous screening.

Cost-Effectiveness Analysis: Results

Mortality-Based Results

The 2-yearly screening programme for women aged 50-70 is expected to detect 26% of all diagnosed breast cancers in the popu-lation. The average tumour size of the screen-detected cancers is small: after the build-up period of screening with a relatively high number of prevalent (large) cancers, 80% of all screen-detected cancers will be smaller than 20 mm or non-invasive. This would be 37% in the non-screening situation. The proportion of women with axillary lymph-node metastases is approximately 60% of the proportion in clinically diagnosed cases, given the same tumour size. The start of the screening programme will initially result in a sharp rise in the number of newly diagnosed cases, with a maximum increase of 17% (1,450 cancers) in the year 1993. From 1996 onwards, the total number of diagnosed breast cancers will increase by 3.5% each year, compared to the expected situation without screening.

Earlier diagnosis will gradually reach its impact on mortality reduction. After 10 years the number of women who will die from breast cancer may have fallen from 3,675 to 3,325. A maximum annual reduction in breast cancer mortality of 16% (700 women) in the total population is attainable from 2015 onwards. On average, each year of screening will prevent 630 breast cancer deaths, leading to a total of 17,000 within a 27-year programme (Table 2). The total costs for screening are 300 million US dollars and the additional costs of treating and following up more women earlier are 72 million (5% discount rate). Inversely, a large decrease in the cost is expected for women with advanced breast cancer (-128 million). The net additional cost of 233 million US dollars divided by 61,000 life-years gained results in a CE ratio of 3,825 US dollars per life-year gained (5% discount rate).

Quality of Life and Cost-Utility

Table 2 shows favourable and unfavourable effects of screening. The numbers relate to the total programme over the whole period of the screening programme (1990-2017) and the average numbers per million total female population per year of screening.

Although mortality reduction is the fundamental endpoint, there is much debate about other desirable and undesirable consequences of screening that may influence quality of life. We, therefore, combined the

Table 2. A review of favourable and unfavourable effects of breast cancer screening in the Netherlands, 1990-2017 (2-yearly screening between the ages of 50 and 70)*

	Total number	Per million women per year
Favourable effects		
Fewer breast cancer deaths	17,000	84
Life-years gained	260,000	1,284
Less treatment advanced disease	17,000	84
Fewer adjuvant therapies	8,300	41
Fewer breast amputations	11,900	59
Fewer biopsies outside screening	50,500	249
Unfavourable effects		
Screening investigations	15,800,000	78,024
Lead time life-years with breast cancer	275,000	1,258
Negative biopsies	33,000	163
More surgical treatments	9,200	45
More radiation treatments	10,300	51

* see also [7]

changes in life expectancy with the expected changes in morbidity. The large increase in women-years in follow-up is almost entirely responsible for the negative quality of life adjustment, whereas the decrease in the number of advanced breast cancer patients as a result of screening accounts for 70% of the positive quality of life adjustment. In the 27-year programme, a total of 252,000 Quality-Adjusted Life-Years (QALYs) are gained, which represents a slight decrease compared to non-adjusted life-years gained (260,000). Since the most favourable effects are preceded by unfavourable effects, this difference grows if effects and costs are discounted. The cost-utility ratio is 5.6% higher than the cost-effectiveness ratio, i.e., 4,050 US dollars per QALY gained (Table 3).

Table 3. Effects on mortality, costs, cost-effectiveness and cost-utility for different breast cancer screening policies (1990-2017) in the Netherlands. Five percent discount rate and costs in million US dollars (unless stated). Cost amounts are expected differences between situation with and without screening

Age group Screening interval	50-70 2 years	40-70 2 years	50-75 2 years	50-65 3 years
Breast cancer deaths prevented*	17,000	17,800	19,450	10,800
Life-years gained*	260,000	290,000	275,000	180,000
Cost of screening	300	457	310	185
Cost of assessment/biopsy	-10	-62	2	-12
Cost of primary treatment	50	57	71	26
Cost of follow-up	22	25	27	14
Cost of advanced disease	-128	-131	-145	-80
Difference in costs	233	346	265	133
Breast cancer deaths prevented	6,000	6,115	6,790	3,770
Life-years gained	61,000	64,000	64,500	41,000
Quality-adjusted Life-years gained (QALY)	57,500	59,500	59,500	39,300
Cost per life-year gained (CE ratio)	3,825	5,385	4,100	3,235
Cost per QALY	4,050	5,815	4,450	3,400

* not discounted

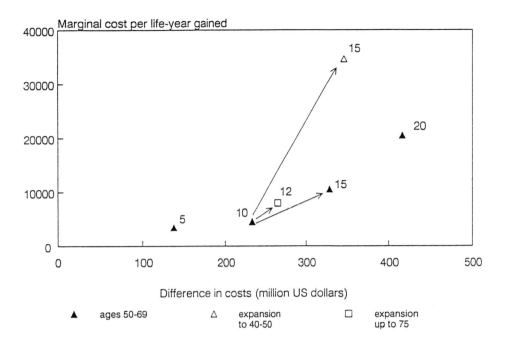

Fig. 2. Marginal cost-effectiveness (additional US dollars per additional life-years gained) of 6 breast cancer screening policies: 5, 10, 15 or 20 invitations in the age group 50-70, 12 invitations in the age group 50-75 and 5 invitations during ages 40-49 followed by 10 invitations during ages 50-70. The corresponding differences in cost for each screening policy have been put at the horizontal axis. Five percent discount rate

Alternative Screening Policies

Two important questions regarding screening policies are frequently discussed. The first is whether or not to extend the programmes to younger age groups. In Table 3, the second column shows a 50% increase in the cost of 2-yearly screening for women aged 40-70, compared to that for women aged 50-70. Using the Kopparberg/Ostergötland-trial estimate for the 40-50 group, the total number of prevented breast cancer deaths increases by 800, which only corresponds to a 5% increase in the discounted number of life-years gained. The difference in costs is strongly influenced by our assumption that assessment procedures outside the programme will diminish in proportion to the decrease in clinically diagnosed breast cancer cases as a result of screening. Applying this assumption to the young screening group, the relatively high number of medical procedures at present in the under-fifties results in a 6-fold higher savings in cost of assessment than in the principal policy despite a lower positive predictive value. The CE ratio is 40% higher

than with 2-yearly screening starting at age 50.

The extra cost per additional life-year gained, marginal CE ratio, when comparing 2-yearly screening in the age group 40-70 with 2-yearly screening in the age group 50-70, is 35,000 US dollars. This may be compared with the option of more intensive screening within the age group 50-70 (15 invitations), with an expected marginal CE ratio of only 10,550 US dollars per additional life-year gained (Fig. 2).

The second question is whether screening should continue in women older than 70. In the age group 70-75 both the attendance rate for screening and women's life-expectancy are decreasing, but the incidence and mortality rates for breast cancer and the sensitivity of mammography are relatively high. Two additional screens up to the age of 75 would increase both the number of prevented breast cancer deaths and costs by approximately 15%. The CE ratio is only 7% higher compared to the principal policy, and the cost-utility ratio 10% (Table 3). The relatively lower number of life-years gained per death prevented in the 70+ group, when compared to the 50-70 group, results in a marginal CE of 8,000 US dollars per additional life-year gained (Fig. 2). However, this is definitely more favourable than extension to younger age groups and compares well with intensifying the programme within the age group 50-70.

The final column in Table 3 shows that a longer screening interval as in the UK-policy is also relatively cost-effective: it would result in a CE ratio of 3,235 US dollars per life-year gained in the Dutch situation. The additional costs are 57% and the life-years gained amount to 68% of those in the present Dutch programme.

Influence of Other Variables

The accuracy of our CE ratios may be influenced by a large number of factors of which the possible improvement in prognosis is certainly the most crucial [7]. Table 4 summarises 8 other factors, which appear to ac-count for more than a 5% difference in CE ratio, if varied within plausible ranges. The only variable for which our estimate may well have resulted in too high a predicted CE ratio for the principal policy is the cost for women with advanced breast cancer. We have used a moderate average cost estimate per treatment [14]. Future treatment modalities will definitely increase the costs, which could result in higher predicted savings due to screening.

The positive predictive value of the mammographic screening test and the possible change in attitude of women in the screening interval appear to be important factors to be monitored right from these first years of implementation. If we assume that mass screening would only reduce the present 33% of assessment procedures known or registered as "for preventive reasons", the CE ratio increases by 18% to 4,465 US dollars per life-year gained. If implementing a programme for women aged 50 and over were to lead to a significant increase in the demand for mam-

Table 4. Alternative assumptions, other than mortality reduction, which influence the cost-effectiveness of 2-yearly mammographic screening of women aged 50-70 (CE in US$ per life-year gained)

	Actual data or assumption in principal variant	Alternative assumption	CE ratio and % difference with principal variant
Cost for treatment of advanced breast cancer	US$ 21,000/woman	25% higher costs	3,300 (- 14%)
Capacity of screening units	12,000 women/year	10,000/year/unit	4,100 (+ 7%)
Positive predictive value of mammographic screening test	51% on average over all rounds	43%	4,130 (+ 8%)
Follow-up examinations of treated women	every 3 months in first 2 years	twice as frequent	4,190 (+ 9%)
Total costs of screening	US$ 40/screen	US$ 43	4,225 (+10%)
Non-medical direct costs	not included	include travel, time and out of pocket costs women	4,460 (+17%)
Demands for mammograms outside screening programme	decrease in assessment proportional to decrease clinical cancers	only decrease in assessment for preventive reasons	4,465 (+18%)
Indirect costs	not included	include medical costs for other diseases in life-years gained	7,259 (+90%)

mograms in the group of women under 50, CE could also deteriorate considerably.

The most influential direct cost components are the cost of follow-up procedures, due to the variability of the protocols for treated breast cancer patients, and the cost of screening. The latter may, for various reasons, become higher than expected when the national programme is under way. With present uncertainties a 10% increase in costs and CE in the Netherlands could be forecast. Time and other non-medical expenses, including travel, for the women involved increase by 17% the CE for 2-yearly screening in the age group 50-70. In particular, the inclusion of indirect costs (production losses and additional costs due to other diseases in the life-years gained) would double the CE ratio. However, these variants may only be compared with the cost-effectiveness ratios of other health-care programmes if those ratios are calculated in the same way.

Discussion

Two-yearly mammograhic screening for women aged 50-70 is expected to reduce breast cancer mortality by 16% in the Dutch population. At the same time, this attainable reduction is also the main uncertainty in calculating the balance between effects and costs for breast cancer screening. Variation of other assumptions generally results in CE ratios ranging from 3,000 to 5,000 US dollars per life-year, or 3,200 to 5,300 US dollars per QALY gained. To our knowledge, no superior cost-utility ratios have yet been reported for other cancer screening programmes. This is even true if an immediate 25% improvement in survival of breast cancer cases is assumed, irrespective of screening.

Differences in QALYs is a more preferable measure than crude life-years gained alone. When taking into account associated morbidity for all possible phases, other favourable and unfavourable effects besides mortality reduction have only limited impact and appear to cancel each other out. More extreme assumptions on the expected utilities in the different phases result in an adjustment of be-

tween -19% (most unfavourable) and +3% (most favourable) on life-years gained for 2-yearly screening of women aged 50-70 [16]. Our evaluation of the effect on quality of life strongly supports the decision to introduce mammographic screening for women aged 50 and over.

Programmes with a screening interval of 2 or 3 years are both relatively cost-effective. If the budget is restricted, a 3-year interval might be appropriate. Quality of life appears of minor influence.

At present, nationwide screening for women under 50 is not to be recommended. Controversy on the effectiveness of screening in this group is strong, but all recent publications and trials suggest that there is no short-term benefit in terms of mortality reduction. Our analysis shows that the assumption of a possible, slight reduction still leads to a very unfavourable balance in terms of marginal cost-effectiveness and cost-utility. A 1.5-year screening interval is often advocated in this age group in order to minimise the relatively high number of interval cancers [17]. From a CE point of view, considering the present estimates on mortality reduction, it would further deteriorate the unfavourable balance between life-years gained and costs. Except for the HIP-trial, there are no other data on which to base a favourable long-term estimate. Moreover, it appeared that this younger age group is, as in other countries, already undergoing mammographic examinations too often. Implementation of screening for women aged 50 and over may catalyse the demand for "screening" in younger age groups even further [18], which would be regarded as a negative side effect of screening women aged 50 and over.

Comparing the predictions in our CE analysis with (very) early outcome measures will have to serve as an early check on the effectiveness of the Dutch nationwide programme. In the Netherlands, 3 centres have now formed such a national evaluation team and a national expert and training centre is responsible for quality control regarding mammography and pathology. Possible unfavourable effects such as large regional differences in treatment or the mentioned increase in mammograhies for younger women have to be excluded as much as possible. The present analysis will, to a large extent, form the basis for national screening evaluations. It has also pinpointed some aspects that are not directly related to the screening performances, but may strongly influence the CE of the programme or the women's quality of life. We will continue our research on the demand for mammograms outside screening and the possibility of a survival improvement irrespective of screening. Furthermore, we are engaged in research on costs and effects of breast cancer screening in other (European) countries. In conclusion, the implementation of breast cancer screening programmes for women aged 50 and older with a 2 or 3-year interval should be further stimulated, provided that a high mammographic and staff quality is guaranteed and that a high level of national assessment is realised.

Conclusions on the Use of CE Analysis

A cost-effectiveness analysis as described in this chapter is a useful addition to other research in the field of cancer screening. Some of the advantages are the following:

1. Perhaps its most important function is that it serves as an integrative framework. Seemingly disparate facts can be related to each other and discussion between different disciplines involved in screening is stimulated.
2. A cost-effectiveness analysis may reveal gaps in knowledge which have to be filled in order to evaluate screening properly. In this way, applied research can be proposed that completes these gaps most efficiently.
3. The relationship between social costs of a programme and population health effects is explored in detail. Only in this way can health services ultimately be compared in order to choose the socially most desirable package of services.
4. By making detailed predictions over the years to come, an important ingredient for a future monitoring system is provided.

The uniform approach to evaluation in the cost-effectiveness study makes a comparison between different health-care services possible. In the long run, this will enhance a more rational approach to decision making in health care.

REFERENCES

1   Warner KE, Luce BR: Cost-benefit and cost-effectiveness analysis in health care. Health Administration Press, Ann Arbor 1982
2   Drummond MF, Stodddart GL, Torrance GW: Methods for the economic evaluation of health care programmes. Oxford University Press, Oxford 1987
3   Habbema JDF, van Oortmarssen GJ, Lubbe JThN et al: The MISCAN simulation program for the evaluation of screening for disease. Comput Meth Progr Biomed 1984 (20):79-93
4   Habbema JDF, Lubbe JTh N, van Oortmarssen GJ et al: A simulation approach to cost-effectiveness and cost benefit calculations of screening for early detection of disease. Eur J Oper Res 1987 (29):159-166
5   Habbema JDF, de Koning HJ: Breast cancer screening in the Netherlands. In: Greberman M, Prorock PC and Shapiro S (eds) Proceedings of the December 1988 Workshop on Information Systems in Breast Cancer Detection. 1991
6   van der Maas PJ, de Koning HJ, van Ineveld BM et al: The cost-effectiveness of breast cancer screening. Int J Cancer 1989 (43):1055-1060
7   de Koning HJ, van Ineveld BM, van Oortmarssen GJ, de Haes JCJM, Collette HJA, Hendriks JHCL, van der Maas PJ: Breast cancer screening and cost-effectiveness; policy alternatives, quality of life considerations and the possible impact of uncertain factors. Int J Cancer 1991 (49):531-537
8   de Koning HJ, van Ineveld BM, van Oortmarssen GJ et al: The costs and effects of mass screening for breast cancer (in Dutch). Final Report Erasmus University Rotterdam, 1990
9   Habbema JDF, Lubbe JThN, van der Maas PJ et al: A computer simulation approach to the evaluation of mass screening. MEDINFO-83. In: Van Bemmel JH, Bal MJ, Wigertz O (eds). North-Holland, Amsterdam 1983 pp 1222-1225
10 Tabár L, Fagerberg G, Duffy SW et al: The Swedish two county trial of mammographic screening for breast cancer: recent results and calculation of benefit. J Epidemiol Comm Hlth 1989 (43):107-114
11 Andersson I, Aspegren K, Janzon L et al: Mammographic screening and mortality from breast cancer: the Malmö mammographic screening trial. Br Med J 1988 (297):943-948
12 van Oortmarssen GJ, Habbema JDF, van der Maas PJ et al: A model for breast cancer screening. Cancer 1990 (66):1601-1612
13 de Koning HJ, van Oortmarssen GJ, van Ineveld BM et al: Breast cancer screening: its impact on clinical medicine. Br J Cancer 1990 (61):292-297
14 de Koning HJ, van Ineveld BM, de Haes JCJM, van Oortmarssen GJ, Klijn JGM, van der Maas PJ: Advanced breast cancer and its prevention by screening. Br J Cancer 1992 (65):950-955
15 Russel LB: Evaluating preventive care. The Brooking Institute, Washington 1987
16 de Haes JCJM, de Koning HJ, van Oortmarssen GJ, van Agt HME, de Bruyn AE, van der Maas PJ: The impact of a breast cancer screening programme on quality-adjusted life-years. Int J Cancer 1991 (49):538-544
17 Tabár L, Fagerberg G, Day NE, Holberg L: What is the optimum interval between mammographic screening examinations? An analysis based on the latest results of the Swedish two-county breast cancer screening trial. Br J Cancer 1987 (55):547-551
18 Ashby J, Buxton M, Gravelle H: Will a breast cancer screening programme change the workload and referral practice of general practitioners? J Epidemiol & Comm Hlth 1990 (44):36-38

Programme Organisation in Breast Cancer Screening

Barbara A. Thomas

Clinical Director, Jarvis Screening and National Training Centre, Guildford, Surrey GU1 1JL, United Kingdom

Programme organisation depends upon the constraints imposed by the resources available. The prevailing attitudes both of the medical profession and of the women to be screened may influence some aspects of programme planning, so that organisational details may not be readily transferable between countries. In general, a population screening programme will need initial capitalisation in terms of equipment and premises (centralised or mobile units) together with investment in the training of suitable personnel. An early decision is required to clarify whether the organisation and management of the programme will be undertaken as an extension of a hospital-based radiology department or whether it will fall within the responsibility of the public health or non-acute community services.

Planning needs to begin at least one year before the start of the screening programme. Early decisions need to be taken with regard to the population to be screened, the screening procedure itself and the evaluation of women with screen-detected abnormalities and implications for their treatment. Only subsequently can detailed plans be made (Table 1).

The Population to be Screened

Most programmes concentrate breast cancer screening upon a target population defined by age alone, no risk factor having yet been proved sufficiently specific to include the majority of women likely to develop breast cancer within a minority of the female population. Since no programme to date has shown convincing evidence of population breast cancer mortality reduction as a consequence of screening women below the age of 50, service screening is usually concentrated above that age. The choice of an upper age limit will depend not only upon epidemiological considerations but also on practical issues such as a lower attendance rate among older women and a balance between the use of resources to include a wider age range as against more frequent screening.

Table 1. Organisational timetable

Decisions to be made by one year before screening is to start:

1. Determine the target population
2. Decide the method of identification of individuals within the target population, preferably establish access to an age/sex register
3. Determine the screening modality to be used
4. Decide the re-screening interval
5. Calculate the proposed annual screening workload
6. Consider the computerisation requirements for the programme (hardware and software)
7. Consider policies for the subsequent evaluation of women with screen-detected abnormalities and their treatment
8. Identify the financial resources required and available for the programme

---

Most programmes consider 65 or 70 to be a suitable upper age limit, on the assumption that a normal mammogram at that age makes death from a clinically presenting subsequent carcinoma unlikely within the following decade, after which the probability of an alternative cause of death rises sharply. National statistics will provide a guideline as to when the increasing incidence of breast cancer in older women is considered to be balanced by the decreasing proportion of deaths from the disease.

Identification of the Individual Women to be Screened

An age/sex register is essential, preferably in a computerised form. Population screening is difficult in the absence of such a register. The accuracy of this register will have important practical repercussions in the invitation of women to come forward for screening.

The Screening Modality

For women older than 50, mammography has to date proven the most sensitive method for the detection of the smaller breast cancers and will be included in any screening programme. The addition of a clinical examination may be requested by those not familiar with modern mammography and, should it be adopted, has major financial consequences. For this age group, the marginal costs of the addition of a clinical examination are not usually justified by a significant increase in the detection of non-invasive and stage I breast cancers. If mammography is the sole screening modality, a decision will be required as to whether one or two mammographic views are taken. While the 30% mortality reduction shown in the Swedish Two-Counties trial was obtained using single-view mammography, many radiologists feel that for the initial screening examination a 45° medio-lateral oblique supplemented by a cranio-caudal view is preferable. It is argued that the second view will increase sensitivity and specificity, thereby reducing the number of women who require evaluation of screen-detected abnormalities at the next stage in the procedure. As regards symptomatic women, more cancers are visualised with two views than with a single mammographic view but there is no conclusive evidence that this is applicable in the screening situation. Early results from the British Programme appear to show a similar detection rate between centres using one view and two views at the expense of a slightly higher recall rate with single-view mammography (1-2%). This is a problem which needs addressing at the training level if one-view mammography is used since decision-making on one film alone is not a normal part of radiological procedure. If resources are finite for a given budget or staffing level, it appears that around 50% more women can be screened for the same resources, using a single rather than two views. There may be greater benefit from screening more women with a single view, and this may possibly allow a wider age range while using the same resources.

Though radiation exposure is minimal with optimum technique, the normal woman will receive twice the radiation from two-view mammography as compared with single view. There is more general agreement that for subsequent screening examinations a single view may be employed for the majority of women.

Those planning screening programmes are advised to visit units using both single and two-view mammography before making a decision. In a 7-hour working day, two radiographers using one piece of mammographic equipment may be expected to comfortably screen 70 women by single-view mammography, allowing a short time to interview the women in order to obtain information relevant to the interpretation of the mammograms, elicit any current symptoms and answer their queries. Assuming a 70% acceptance rate, it is usual to invite around 100 women per day per mammographic unit staffed by two radiographers. Using two views, the same radiographers may be expected to screen approximately 50 women. Therefore, there will probably be implications for staffing levels, training requirements, and numbers of mammographic units resting upon this decision.

The Re-screening Interval

Different countries, with different medico-political systems, when considering the same evidence from screening trials, have come to different conclusions regarding the re-screening interval. An interval shorter than one year seems impractical and intervals between 18 months and 3 years are commonly used with two years being the most frequent choice for mammographic breast cancer screening.

At this point it should be possible to calculate the number of women to be invited for screening each year and how many screening units would be required for the primary screen if all eligible women were to attend. The actual workload will depend upon the acceptance rate. Since requirements will differ, if 90% of the women are likely to attend as compared with 60-70%, a feasibility study in the appropriate district is desirable, but otherwise an approximate indication may be taken from the proportion of the population who vote in a general election. In the UK, estimates were based upon a 70% acceptance rate which has proved realistic overall. There is an apparent trend for acceptance rates to be higher in rural districts and lower in large urban conurbations, though this may be partially explained by less accurate age/sex registers for the more mobile urban population.

Screening Workload

When age range, screening method and frequency have been agreed and acceptance rate estimated, it is possible to establish the annual workload which will be generated by the programme. The size of a working unit may be determined on the basis of geography, population, the maximisation of use of screening equipment, e.g., mammogram machines or availability of personnel. Calculations must be made of the capital and establishment requirements and of the ongoing revenue costs and staff needed to implement the programme. When calculating the workload of a unit, it must be appreciated that the staff need to be specifically trained in this field and that locum staff to cover holidays or sickness are usually unavailable at the commencement of a programme. Schedules based upon a 40-week year usually allow sufficient leeway to cover these eventualities. In a situation where 10,000 women are to be screened annually, experience shows that if plans are made to screen 200 weekly it is unlikely that after two or 3 years the screening schedule will be on target; if, however, facilities are organised so as to screen 250 women weekly, it will be possible to adhere to annual schedules while decreasing screening activity for holiday periods, staff sickness and continued training but maintaining the appropriate annual screening throughput.

Computerisation Requirements

A large volume of data is generated by any screening programme and decisions need to be taken concerning the choice of computer hardware and software for all but the smallest programmes. Computer hardware needs careful selection: not only the volume of data needs consideration but the speed of access becomes important in the daily running of the programme. Software may need to be written specifically for the programme or a suitable system may be commercially available. Advice should be sought both from computer specialists and from those already using breast screening computer programmes.

Subsequent Evaluation of Women with Screen-Detected Abnormalities and their Treatment

Following the primary screening procedure, there are 3 different strategies for the management of women having a possible abnormality (Table 2).

Option I: Swedish Two-Counties

Women are recalled to the primary screening unit where 3-view mammography is carried out. Films are subsequently read centrally

Table 2. Options following primary screening

I	II	III
e.g., Swedish Two-Counties	e.g., the UK	e.g., The Netherlands
↓ If ?	↓ If ?	↓ If ?
Recall for a 3-view mammography at the site of primary screen	Recall for assessment, i.e., second stage screen for full evaluation at a specialist centre	Advice to the woman's own doctor to arrange hospital referral to a specialist of the doctor's choice
↓ If still ?	↓ If cancer or still ?	
Recall to central unit for full evaluation	Surgical biopsy / treatment	
↓ If cancer or still ?		
Surgical biopsy / treatment		

and if carcinoma cannot be excluded, then the woman is recalled again for full evaluation where facilities for specialist mammographic techniques are available together with clinical examination, needle biopsy and, increasingly, ultrasound. If in-patient biopsy is still required to establish a diagnosis or treatment is indicated, appropriate arrangements may then be made at this visit, or a further visit to see a surgeon may be required prior to admission. The advantage of this system is that if screening takes place in remote country districts, fewer women need to make the long journey to the specialist centre for evaluation, as their query will have been settled by 3-view mammography. In many instances, however, this gives no opportunity for discussion with the woman of the reason for recall, or for personal reassurance when all is well. Applicability will depend on the acceptance of this by the women concerned as well as on the location of the screening unit in relation to the evaluation unit.

Option II: The United Kingdom

Evaluation of screen-detected abnormalities is considered to be an integral part of the screening procedure and is centrally organised and agreed before the primary screen is carried out. Women are recalled to specialist clinics, usually staffed by the same screening radiologists who are responsible for the interpretation of the primary screening films as well as by specialists with clinical and cytological expertise. Facilities are available for specialised mammographic techniques to be carried out as well as clinical examination, ultrasound, and needle biopsy of palpable and impalpable lesions. In some cases, it is possible to make arrangements for admission for surgical biopsy or treatment at the time of the visit, should this be indicated; in others, treatment may be carried out nearer the woman's home by local surgeons. This option ensures specialist evaluation for all women together with the opportunity to discuss the reason for their recall, give the results, and provide counselling when appropriate.

In either of these options, it is essential to minimise the number of women in whom malignancy cannot be fully excluded but the degree of suspicion is insufficient to justify surgical biopsy. Such women may need to be screened or re-evaluated before the next routine screen is due. These women can be accommodated at the evaluation level as the programme progresses since fewer women are recalled from the primary screen at screening visits after the first.

Option III: The Netherlands

The screening programme carries responsibility only for the primary screening mammogram and when any possible abnormality is detected, the woman is referred to her own doctor who may arrange referral to the hospital of his choice. Success is dependent upon the doctor choosing a specialist evaluation team appropriate to the abnormality suspected and in many instances will separate screening from evaluation expertise.

In all options, there is the recommendation, actual or implied, that non-palpable disease is best evaluated and treated in specialist breast units. Local medical practice may be important in ensuring the acceptability of whichever option is chosen and this should be discussed by all medical personnel involved. In countries where the woman has her own personal medical practitioner, the support of that doctor is crucial. Without this the woman may be referred for further evaluation of screen-detected abnormalities to units which do not have the appropriate facilities and expertise and substitute for these an unacceptably high biopsy rate.

The End of the Screening Process Needs Definition

In option III the end of the screening process is reached after the first films are interpreted. In options I and II, it is reached when a diagnosis of cancer is made or an equivocal situation requires surgical biopsy. At this point the woman ceases to be a client and becomes a patient within the normal medical services of the country. A clear break at this point may be helpful when organising the financial aspects of the programme, even though in some cases the treating surgeon may also be a member of the evaluation team.

Treatment Implications

When a screening programme has been running for some years and is established in the re-screening phase, there should be no greater treatment implications than prior to screening, though the stage of the disease may be expected to be much more favourable. There should be less requirement for treatment relating to terminal disease balanced by an increase in the number of localisation procedures required prior to surgery. Special needs concerning the histological examination of surgical specimens must be considered since large tissue sections or large numbers of small blocks may need to be examined. This is much more time consuming than the examination of a clinical breast lump specimen. Treatment policies for in-situ disease and well-differentiated low grade small invasive tumours are desirable, but there is, as yet, no generally agreed policy for treatment of these lesions and the establishment of clinical trials must be considered.

Arrangements to be Made 6-12 Months Before Screening Commences

During this period much work is needed to finalise the details of the screening procedure. Preliminary discussions are required concerning the invitation to participate, the provision of facilities for screening in terms of venue, procedure, equipment and staffing, data collection and quality assurance measures.

Certain key personnel will need to be appointed so that they may be involved in the planning stages of their own programmes.

The Screening Procedure

The Invitation to Participate

The ideal means of ensuring that an invitation reaches every eligible woman is a continuously updated, accurate age/sex register. This is rarely available and some form of accuracy check immediately prior to screening may be necessary.

Attention should be paid to the form of the invitation, whether it is an actual appointment which may be changed if inconvenient, or merely an invitation to apply for an appointment. Pilot studies indicate a higher uptake when an appointment is given rather than a request to apply for one. The appropriate letters will need to be designed and agreed between those organising the programme and those who may be concerned in the medical supervision of the women, e.g., the general practitioners.

Procedures should be agreed to maximise acceptance rates. These would normally include a policy for the distribution of information about the screening programme both to the women and the medical profession. This may necessitate the education of medical practitioners and other medical and paramedical personnel, working both within the community and the hospital fields, in relation to the reasons for implementing screening and how it is to be carried out. General publicity about the screening programme has to be carefully planned, particularly if screening activity is confined within relatively small localities at any one time, since inappropriate requests for screening at unscheduled times can cause illwill and decrease the eventual acceptance rate. A policy for non-responders is required: will further contact be made, and if so, when, by whom and what form will it take?

Provision of Facilities

Location of Screening Unit

Screening may be carried out in a permanent building which may additionally provide the centre for the evaluation of screen-detected abnormalities and/or for the organisation of the programme; alternatively, screening may be carried out by mobile units. The choice will largely depend upon geographical factors, a large city population often being best served by a unit in or near the major shopping centre while a scattered rural population is commonly screened by a mobile unit, possibly sited in the local market town. If mobile units are used, they need careful design both with reference to the radiographic facilities, the working conditions of those staffing them and the problems associated with site preparation and unit moves. Expenses will be required for staff travelling and if the unit is sited some distance from base, then either the radiographers will have a shorter working time for screening activity (may need more units and staff), or overtime payments or time off in lieu will have financial consequences which must be considered at the planning stage.

Quality control of the radiography is essential and processing is, by many, considered to be best carried out at the central unit where quality control measures are routine. Processing on mobile units is possible but needs careful daily quality assurance measures. Such procedures are used in Holland whereas in the United Kingdom it is more usual to have central processing. It is not easy to move these mobile units on a daily basis if high quality is to be maintained, and it is suggested that prepared sites are used with the appropriate electrical facilities laid on, so as to avoid the use of separate generators. Should these have to be used, it should be possible to separate them from the mobile unit when in action as there could be problems with vibration and noise. If mobile units are considered, advice should be sought from those with practical experience of their use in the field.

Equipment

The radiologist and superintendent radiographer for the programme need to be consulted at the planning stage when the layout of the rooms or interior of the mobile unit and choice of equipment are being decided upon.

Screening Procedure

Careful decisions need to be taken concerning the details of the screening procedure. The amount of information elicited from the woman should be that minimal amount necessary to interpret the films. If epidemiological data is required for research purposes, this represents an additional cost above that of screening because of the time taken to elicit such information.

It should be decided what information should be given to the women at the screening visit. This should include as a minimum an indication of when she may expect to hear the results, what procedure is likely to be followed if a clear result cannot be given, and when she is likely to be screened next. The "normal" letter should include the information that though mammography is the most sensitive test currently available, it does not guarantee the detection of all breast cancers which may be present. Advice as to what she should do and whom she should consult in case she notices any specified breast symptoms, is also desirable.

Staffing

Two radiographers are suggested as basic staffing for each mammogram screening unit as they can both obtain information from the woman and carry out the screening procedure. If one of them is replaced by a clerk or nurse, she can only perform a small part of the screening procedure and the woman would always therefore meet two members of the staff in a short period of time and may not have sufficient opportunity to establish a relationship with either. Should a radiographer unexpectedly not be available on a certain day, e.g., because of illness, there is no way that a clerk could carry out the screening pro-

cedure, but if the unit is normally staffed by two radiographers, it is possible to proceed with one radiographer and an additional nurse or clerk sent out from the central unit to help with the non-radiographic work in an emergency.

Processing and Film Interpretation

Arrangements must be considered for the transfer of processed films from a mobile to the central unit for interpretation or for the transport in light-tight containers of exposed films for processing centrally. Quality control measures for processing need to be agreed. The handling of developed films and their correlation with paperwork and/or computer information has staffing implications. Radiographers may process and handle films; the advantage being that they see their own films regulary. Alternatively, dark-room technicians or clerical staff may be employed for some of this work but this alternative has the disadvantage that they cannot replace the radiographers in the screening programme in an emergency. Viewing conditions for interpretation must be considered. It is usual to load batches of films onto multiple viewers and some 70-80 sets of films are generally read at one sitting, representing one day's work for two radiographers. It takes about one hour to load such a batch of films and 1 to 1.5 hours for an experienced viewer to interpret them. A decision is required as to whether the screening films will be single or double read. The second pair of eyes probably adds around 10% to the detection rate even with experienced viewers. After interpretation the films need to be removed, data entered into the computing system, unless there is automatic input to the computer by the film reader, and the normal films filed away. A fail-safe mechanism is required to ensure that women who should be recalled are actually recalled and the files of these women may advantageously be separated from those of "normal" women at this point. On the re-screening visits, previous films need to be available for comparison and preferably loaded for automatic viewing together with those of the current screen.

Filing

Facilities for storage and retrieval are required. The possibility of women retaining their own films has not been used in large programmes. The cost of packing and posting them may well exceed the storage costs and this option poses additional problems of lost or forgotten films at subsequent screens.

Data Collection and Quality Assurance Measures

Documentation and letters need to be designed and linked with the proposed computerisation system. It may be possible in some circumstances to dispense with paperwork and work directly on computer terminals. If this is done, there may be medico-legal consequences of being unable to produce a contemporarily written record unless there is some mechanism by which alterations in the computer database can be recorded. There is also limitation of the venue at which any records can be made or work carried out as well as the impossibility of working when there is any downtime with the computer system.

Quality assurance measures are desirable at all stages of the screening programme, not merely for the radiographic aspects and these need discussion at an early stage, particularly as there are organisational and financial consequences. Discussion of measures to be taken if previously agreed standards are not reached is essential, as is the nomination of someone to take responsibility for ensuring that the appropriate action be taken.

The overall success of the programme will eventually be measured by any change in breast cancer mortality within the population offered screening. This entails monitoring the breast cancers in the population as a whole and the establishment of an accurate cancer registry is highly desirable. Some form of cancer identification unit working in conjunction with the screening programme, the general practitioners, the hospital's surgical, pathological and radiotherapeutic services as well as monitoring of the local death returns is needed to liaise with the cancer registry and to secure the inclusion of all cases. Earlier measures of success relate to the screening programme parameters themselves and additionally, the identification of and estimated prognosis for interval cancers and cancers in women who fail to attend for screening. The establishment of a cancer registry or other cancer identification unit of high accuracy is expensive. This factor needs consideration at the commencement of any proposed screening programme.

The Appointment of Key Personnel

The programme director or manager, the financial adviser, radiologist and superintendent radiographer should ideally be appointed about 6 months before the programme is due to start so that they may have the opportunity to choose equipment and plan detailed procedures before the actual screening starts. They will also be closely involved in the appointment of other staff.

The Last 6 Months Before Screening

Key personnel should already be in post and decisions should have been taken regarding major aspects of the screening programme. The first 3 months of this period will be occupied by the procedures necessary for the appointment of virtually the whole staff who will be required for the programme, the preparation of buildings or mobile units and the ordering and installation of equipment.

Staffing

Recruitment procedures for the employment of professional staff may be lengthy and consideration must be given to the possibility of a 3 months' notice being required by the previous employer before staff appointed may join the unit. Other staff may need to give only one month's notice but the advertising of the posts, short listing and interview procedures can take 2 months. Administrative and office staff may be difficult to recruit in some circumstances, particularly if the screening unit is in an area where living expenses are high. During this period the key staff already appointed will be deciding upon the appropriate training courses for new staff and making arrangements for them to attend. Training is required not only for the staff who will be involved with the primary screening procedure but also for those who will deal with the evaluation of women with screen-detected abnormalities. Liaison should be made with those likely to be treating the women from the screening programme, and again further training may be appropriate.

Apart from a working knowledge of the procedures to be followed during the screening programme, specific training outside the unit will be required for the staff listed below.

Medical Staff

Radiologists or other doctors reading screening mammograms will require specific training in this field. It should be pointed out that knowledge of clinical mammography does not provide the appropriate training for the interpretation of screening mammograms. Diagnostic decision-making from films of the symptomatic woman, who commonly has a mass immediately apparent on the mammogram, is quite different from the viewing of 1000 sets of films of breasts with an infinite variety where perhaps 5 among that number may have a malignancy. The subtle signs of the earliest invasive cancers require expertise in the screening field which is acquired by specific training and practice. Up to 3 months' training had been thought to be required initially but recent experience in the United Kingdom has shown that detection rates of over 6 per thousand women first screened in the 50-64 age range may be obtained when the film readers have received a basic short theory course combined with a two-week concentrated and intensive practical experience in a screening training unit. The European Group for Breast Cancer Screening has made recommendations as to the facilities which should be available in such units. Training should not be undertaken too soon since it is desirable that the film readers proceed immediately from their training secondment to reading screening films in their own unit. Careful scheduling is essential and if this ideal timing cannot be achieved, arrangements should, if possible, be made for such a person to see screening films else-

where between training and commencing screening.

Those with previous experience in clinical mammography may sometimes not realise the extent of the variation in normal mammograms and it is essential that they are given the opportunity to view large numbers of normal films, otherwise the minor differences between the two breasts may be too frequently confused with the signs of early malignancy, resulting in a high recall rate. Specificity is very important in the interpretation of screening mammograms.

The full range of quality control procedures essential in a screening programme are not always in routine use in general X-ray departments, and their implementation and control require again specific training. The detection rate of the smallest invasive cancers (less than 1 cm) is generally taken to indicate the quality of the mammography, since the calcifications associated with non-invasive lesions may be more readily seen on suboptimal mammograms.

Radiographers

High-quality mammography is mandatory in any breast cancer screening programme and all screening radiographers need specific training in this field. Courses are required at the theoretical and practical level to ensure correct positioning of the women, especially for the difficult 45° medio-lateral oblique, the basic screening view which should include almost all the breast tissue on the film. These courses should also ensure the establishment of the quality control measures necessary on a daily, weekly and monthly basis. Regular update courses are desirable.

Staff Involved at the Evaluation Stage

The radiologist, clinician and cytopathologist will need specific training concerning the problems of diagnosis of the smallest cancers. Specialist mammographic techniques, ultrasound and the inter-relation between minimal clinical signs and imaging methods need to be explored. Procedures and routines to be followed should be agreed upon and plans should be made for the evaluation of the different types of mammographic abnormality. The appointment of a breast cytopathologist, if not already in post, should be considered. When a presumptive diagnosis of carcinoma has been made, then the expertise needed for the surgical biopsy must be available. Radiological localisation procedures should be familiar to the radiologist and surgeon. The surgeon will need a working knowledge of mammography and should have determined a policy for the treatment of *in-situ* and small invasive carcinomas. Arrangements must be made for specimen radiography when impalpable lesions are excised.

The histopathologist will need further training in those areas of histopathology specifically related to breast cancer screening. There will be a higher proportion of well-differentiated and tubular carcinomas which must be distinguished from radial scar lesions and the problems of *in-situ* disease and epitheliosis with atypia pose problems less commonly met in normal clinical practice. The availability of facilities for the examination of large tissue sections is highly desirable to avoid the time-consuming examination of multiple small sections from many blocks. A frozen section is usually inappropriate for the examination of non-palpable lesions.

Nursing Staff

If nurses are present in the evaluation clinics, they may need to acquire further counselling skills and will need a basic knowledge of the screening programme. Nurse counsellors are desirable for treatment units both to counsel the women in hospital and provide support and advice outside the hospital environment.

Administrative and Office Staff

Familiarisation with the computer system and practice with the use of word processing systems is essential. Training on the extraction of data from the computer system may be required if staff are not familiar with this when appointed. All those involved with answering the telephone or reception work need to be familiar with the questions women commonly ask in these circumstances, and have an-

swers formulated beforehand which have been agreed by the medical and para-medical staff.

Other training requirements will need to be identified as being relevant to individual programmes and the cultural and medical circumstances in which the screening takes place.

The Final 3 Months

Staff will undergo training and the logistics of the invitation system, the screening procedures, the notification of the results and the evaluation of women recalled will be agreed upon and understood by all those who will be involved. The computer system will be tested and final checks on all other equipment will be made.

Documentation will be printed and letters which will be used frequently to convey the same information will be designed.

Publicity

Open meetings for medical, para-medical staff and others, such as health education officers working in related fields, are advisable to give information about the programme. Meetings with those more directly concerned, e.g., general practitioners whose women are to be included in the first stage of the programme, may need to be arranged at the practitioner's home base. All medical and para-medical staff working in the public health field should be aware of the broad principles of the programme and when and where it will take place. General publicity in the newspapers, radio or other media would be appropriate within the locality of the screening programme.

Invitations and Appointments

Appointments or invitations need to be dispatched 3 to 4 weeks before the screening date in order to allow women who may be working to make appropriate arrangements. The names and addresses of the women will therefore need to have been obtained prior to this and the clinics' schedules and appointments given. If evaluation is to be centrally organised, then clinics need to be arranged from one week after the first screening appointment takes place.

Quality assurance measures for the actual process need to have been agreed and radiographic procedures to have been practised. In the meantime, medical staff will have been trained and be informed about the duties they are about to undertake.

Careful planning with adjustments for local reactions and local situations will help the programme to get off the ground smoothly. Continued adjustments will be necessary throughout the life of the programme as there is a continual learning process for all involved. At all stages, much help can be obtained by visiting other well-established screening programmes and instituting the best and most appropriate features seen elsewhere, rather than imitating the details of any particular programme.

It should be appreciated that it is normal for there to be minor problems at this point with buildings, equipment or staff being unavailable at the last minute. Do not be discouraged, you are now ready to screen. All should be well.

Good Luck!

REFERENCES

1   Thomas BA: Medical Fellowship Report, Council of Europe, Secretariat General, Strasbourg. European Breast Cancer Screening Programmes with particular reference to organisation, procedures, further management and treatment. September 1984

2   Breast Cancer Screening. Report to the Health Ministers of England, Wales, Scotland & Northern Ireland by a working group chaired by Professor Sir Patrick Forrest, H.M.S.O. 1986

3   The Costs and Effects of Mass Screening for Breast Cancer. Department of Public Health & Social Medicine, Erasmus Universiteit, Rotterdam. Department of Social Medicine/Department of Radiology, Katholieke Universiteit, Nijmegen. Preventicon/Department of Public Health and Epidemiology, Rijksuniversiteit, Utrecht. Department of Medical Sociology, Rijksuniversiteit, Groningen 1988

4   Cancer Research Campaign Primary Care Education Group: Breast cancer screening - A practical guide for primary care teams. Austoker J. Oxford University Press 1990

5   National Health Service Breast Screening Programme Publications - the U.K. Programme. A series of booklets on many aspects of screening and organisation in the U.K. context. Gray M (ed) National Breast Cancer Screening Education Programme, Department of Community Medicine, Radcliffe Infirmary, Oxford 1990

6   European Group for Breast Cancer Screening: Guidelines for Breast Cancer Screening. Clin Radiol 1987 (38):217
Screening for breast cancer: Recommendations for training. Lancet 1987 (1):398
Screening for breast cancer: Examination and reporting of histopathological preparations. Lancet 1988 (2):953

7   Reports from the various screening trials. See references in Chapter "Screening Trials"

Compliance in Breast Cancer Screening: the Spanish Experience

Nieves Ascunce and Angel Del Moral

Department of Health, Government of Navarra, C/ Conde Oliveto 9, 31002 Pamplona, Spain

Navarra is a region situated to the south of the Western Pyrenees in the North of the Iberian Peninsula. It is an autonomous community with a high degree of self-government within the Spanish State, and has a regional parliament and a government which has full powers in the health sector.

The total population (1986) is 512,512, consisting of 254,786 males and 257,726 females. The population is at zero growth. The population density is only 50 inhabitants per square kilometre: 45,6% in rural areas; 82,8% of urban dwellers live in Pamplona and its surrounding area.

The area comes within the overall public sector of the regional health service.

The Breast Cancer Detection Programme is organised by the government of Navarra in conjunction with the Ministry of Health and the European Community. It includes all women between the ages of 45 and 65 (based on the census). An oblique view screening test of half the breast is carried out every 2 years.

Definition of Compliance

A 100% accrual of any target group is never possible, therefore, in order to achieve the objectives of the screening programme, i.e., reduced mortality, a figure as near to 100% as possible must be sought after.

A low level of compliance implies a new population selection, but in this case not according to a criterion of discrimination on the basis of risk. Women participate by compliance and are not necessarily those with a higher risk of being affected by the disease. Indeed, on many occasions, we have seen that the selection occurs in a negative way, i.e., the women with the lowest risk present themselves, thus causing detection rates in this subgroup to be lower than those estimated for the overall population. At present, the programme is no longer based on population and has effectively become a programme on demand [1].

The question remains as to where the line can be drawn. The difficulty lies in defining this "upper limit of participation" value which is, in consequence, the minimum required for any screening programme. From a public health point of view, it would be the point above which mortality in the target group (both participants and non-participants) drops significantly. Some studies put this figure at 65%.

Below this percentage, benefit can only be seen at an individual level among those participating in the programme, and contradicts thereby the assumption made when implementing it (i.e., that the programme should have benefits on a collective scale).

In attempting to achieve a reduction in the mortality rate, it is obvious that other factors are equally significant: the quality of the mammograph, follow-up of detected suspicions, treatment of confirmed cases, etc. These factors will be analysed in other sections of this chapter.

Sociological Investigation

Those people running the programme will probably know the socio-geographical and human area where it is to be applied. Nevertheless, the view of what is health and sickness in a certain region, conditioned by its anthropological development and cultural influence, may include attitudes (especially among certain groups of people) which make it very difficult to get the message across.

So, to communicate effectively with a given population, it is necessary to investigate the community from a sociological perspective [2] to find out their positive and negative attitudes towards the matter in hand. This will make it easier to understand the circumstances which can better influence reception of the proposals offered.

Our choice of the different types of possible sociological studies [3] was that of groups involving people of similar characteristics. A female psychologist acted as coordinator, introducing the subjects and helping to stimulate group interaction, bringing to light the attitudes which are seen to be normal in that particular social group.

The groups were composed of women from 30-44 and 45-65 years of age from different parts of the region, from different social categories and from both rural and urban areas.

The women under 45 were seen to be better disposed to sickness prevention in general, especially in relation to breast cancer, than their older counterparts. The younger women were familiar with and carried out self-examination, although with a low degree of confidence. They were not highly motivated to attend sessions on the subject. They knew about mammography, and if they did not request it, this was due to the difficulty of getting access to it.

The women in the 45 to 65 age group were poorly informed on preventive methods, and their health concerns were centred on the illness they had suffered. They would not discuss breast cancer spontaneously and preferred to avoid the subject.

These women no longer visit their gynaecologist; only 10% of them knew about mammography, although 50% of those from higher socio-economic groups and in the urban areas had undergone it on their doctor's recommendation.

The campaign, when explained, was seen as having very positive aspects, but the women recognised that they would attend if given a specific appointment. The group of women from rural areas were reluctant to attend and could only be persuasive where easy access was available. It was therefore decided to involve women between 45 and 65 years of age, making them more aware of the risks at that age. The campaign was given a lower emphasis in relation to the younger women. The safety, harmlessness and objectivity of mammography were highlighted.

The sociological study provided us with substantial information on the attitudes and awareness of women, on the need to carry out the programme and on the aspects which should be highlighted in order to achieve a high level of participation. By these means it is hoped that the serious health problem of breast cancer in Navarra will be viewed more optimistically.

Strategy to Stimulate Participation

The need to involve more women led to a major effort throughout the media, in addition to using all those social resources which could contribute to our aims. Furthermore, there is also the need for accessibility to the programme to be guaranteed despite the demand on time and money.

Awareness

The data from the previous sociological study show that there was little interest among women over 45 to undergo a breast examination, this being even more marked over 65 years of age. The vast majority of women of this age also did not know about mammography, and furthermore did not seem worried about breast cancer, or consciously or unconsciously tried to ignore the subject.

All these factors together with the experience of others [4] and our own have led us to the conclusion that in order to achieve 80% of the target population involved in the programme, considerable resources should be mobilised to attain a sufficient level of awareness among the population and encourage women to overcome their initial reluctance to undergo mammography [5].

The basic criteria required to increase awareness were the following:
- the information given had to be true;
- the information should create anxiety, but not dramatically so;
- the information should carry a message of hope that the illness could be beaten;
- the target age range had to be clearly limited;
- the language and images used should be attractive to the whole population;
- health professionals should know and approve the implementation of the programme;
- creating awareness would not only be done through advertising.

All these criteria were duly followed.

As far as mobilisation of social resources was concerned [6], the first moves were designed to obtain a positive committment on the part of medical professionals. In line with the criterion established in Navarra to integrate the activities in the health system, thus avoiding parallel structures, and bearing in mind the influence of the family doctor on many of his women patients, meetings were organised throughout the region with medical personnel and nurses, both from primary care and involved specialisations, to discuss the draft of the programme prior to its approval.

One of the key points in a screening programme is the ability and attitude of health services to cope with the demand generated. To this end, we held several meetings with doctors in breast cancer units in the two-third level hospitals where patients would be sent.

In this way the programme was improved by the suggestions and concerns put forward. Our aim to get a committment from all medical personnel in carrying out the programme was also reinforced.

We are convinced that breast cancer, if detected early enough, can be cured and we want to transmit this conviction to the female population of Navarra. In other words, we aim to reach a "state of opinion" in Navarra regarding breast cancer which means that mammography will become something completely natural for a woman at a certain age.

On the basis of this outlook, all our efforts at enhancing awareness are directed towards providing the woman of 45-65 years of age with an opportunity of doing something for herself in relation to her health, something which, moreover, would be accepted, understood and encouraged by the people close to her and by society at large. With this in mind various activities have been organised with citizens' groups, each one in line with the characteristics of the particular rural or urban area and social structure. In some cases, as in one area on the outskirts of Pamplona, great effectiveness has been achieved by women setting up their own group and appointing people responsible for streets and apartment blocks, thereby achieving complete cooperation. In another (semi-urban) area, the stimulator was a cultural activity group for women. Red Cross volunteers also participated.

These resources have not been sufficiently exploited to date and efforts will continue to endeavour to achieve maximum use of what is available.

The link with a health team is often made through a meeting with an "area health committee", a body in which the public can participate. It includes the local council, trade unions, business, consumer, and residents' associations, etc. This body has always shown great interest and has cooperated actively.

Most of the media have been used to advertise the programme [7], with different forms of presentation in each one. Advertising is always used (planned to appear over various time periods) to achieve complete consistency between the messages and the image based on the previously described criteria. The image should support the idea that although it is directed exclusively at a particular group of women, it does not exclude the rest of the population, especially spouses or children who can contribute (and indeed do so) to encouraging attendance.

All advertising has 4 lines of attack: 1) age limited to 45-65; 2) the risk below this age range is very low; 3) wait for us to call you; answer the call, and 4) prevention means cure.

Given its wide audience and impact, television is the preferred medium to transmit the basic idea of the programme and the 4 messages described above.

Radio has also played an important part in disseminating the messages. Apart from publicity spots, we were able to get a weekly link-up of all the major local radio stations to the screening unit, transmitting messages, advice, criteria, personal experiences, information on the programme of activities, etc. This open phone-in programme reached a wide audience and led to an avalanche of phone calls, not only for on-the-air transmissions but also to the central coordination unit, to ask questions and make a second appointment if they had not attended the first one.

In the press, the use of advertisements with images of the spots and activity programmes is continuous, although different frequency patterns are determined by the area or the level of participation. If the latter drops, advertising is stepped up.

A series of posters has been prepared for those areas where efforts are to be directed, prior to and during the period of appointments.

The public is informed about once every 6 months on the progress of the programme and the results obtained, through press conferences given by the regional health minister. The information is taken up by all the media and the programme receives wide coverage in the form of articles and interviews.

Much time, imagination and money has been spent on this area which accounts for about 20% of the total budget of the programme.

Accessibility

The organisation of the programme is based on the following conditions: decentralisation, free-of-charge services and planned appointments.

Decentralisation

The opinion survey showed that a high level of compliance would only be achieved if the examinations were carried out near the home of the persons called. Two units were established as a result:

A permanent unit in Pamplona, covering women resident in the city and surrounding areas. Various criteria were taken into account so that it could be reached easily: accessibility (centre of Pamplona, well served by bus routes, nearby parking, etc.) and acceptability (a health centre, both primary and specialised, visited regularly by a large number of people). Although the option of installing the unit in a hospital was feasible in terms of space, it was rejected in anticipation of possible refusal by supposedly healthy people to visit a hospital.

A mobile unit which theoretically, on the basis of the accessibility criteria, should visit all places where women of the age range are resident. However, the combination of the efficient use of resources, technical possibilities and, of course, accessibility, led us to a combined system whereby the mobile unit visited medium-sized locations, coinciding with already established health centres in Navarra. In this way, the unit visits localities with enough women of the age range to be able to work for a week, screening about 450 women. We have thereby managed to link the programme into the primary health care network because it has always been set up in a health centre. It can also be used as a waiting room, intermediate point of contact between the coordination unit and the woman, etc. Furthermore, the local population is willing to make the trip to these locations because that is where they normally receive medical care. Nevertheless, we were aware that many women between 45 and 65 years of age do not have their own private means of transport and need somebody else to take them to the health centre. For this reason, a free minibus service was offered to transport the women from each locality (however small) to the mobile unit. The minibus then takes them back to their place of residence. So far, the mobile unit has been installed in 26 localities and the minibus has operated to/from 350 small villages. It has been completely accepted by the target population and has even been used at times when the person in question had her own means of transport.

Free-of-Charge Services

This accessibility should not only be physical but also social and financial [8], i.e., criteria of equity should be applied. It was therefore decided that both screening tests and later diagnostic and treatment stages should be free of charge. Nevertheless, if it is necessary to continue the diagnostic process after the screening test and the woman prefers to go to a private hospital, she is given a copy of her own clinical record. The programme coordination unit contacts the hospital and establishes the follow-up for the patient.

Planned Appointments

The opinion survey initially carried out confirmed all this through direct surveys among the population, similar to the one recently carried out by the European Community as part of the "Europe Against Cancer" programme. It is confirmed that although women recognise that cancer could be avoided, or that they could get an early diagnosis with a higher chance of cure, they do not necessarily take up the means at their disposal. In practice, only a very small proportion of women undergo regular mammographies even though they know that their chances of cure would be greater if they did. For this reason, it is difficult to achieve high levels of coverage through on-demand programmes; the screening programme should actively encourage women to get involved instead of leaving them to take the decision on their own.

Thus, it was agreed that, on the basis of information recorded by the census, the same coordination unit should contact women to request them to attend.

The programme was started up by sending a personalised letter to all women resident in Navarra between the ages of 45 and 65 (the entire target population). The aim of this letter was to explain the programme and advise them that they would be called in for a mammography within 2 years. In this way any women would find out if she were included in the programme or not. These letters were signed by the Regional Health Minister, thus establishing a first contact between himself and the population. This created a new situation for the vast majority of the women.

At a later stage, and in accordance with a previously established schedule, the area of screening was chosen and a second personalised letter was sent inviting the subject to visit the unit and indicating the time and the day reserved for her. Information on the minibus is also included in appointment notices for the mobile unit. In some areas a note from the primary health care team is included, encouraging the woman to attend.

With the aim of producing a positive response on a collective scale, the invitations were sent simultaneously to one particular area (organised by street and apartment block) in such a way that all the residents in that area were allocated the same time.

As it was seen that attendance was high and homogeneous right from the start, it proved unnecessary for the women to confirm their intention to attend. Work was planned on the basis of 85% attendance in rural areas and 75-80% in urban areas.

Although they were recommended to avoid changing their appointment times where possible, all those women who requested an appointment change were received at the most convenient time for them. The administration unit attends to calls during office hours, whereas an answering machine records calls (name, number, reason for calling and caller's telephone number) outside office hours.

While work is being done in the area, the census base is updated. Data is gathered either from women who phone or visit the unit, or from women in the area who attend the programme. The primary care teams involved also participate in this updating process.

Participation is checked daily in order to take further measures if the 65% figure is not reached. These measures include more advertising, contacts with local groups, talks, etc. Should 75% participation not have been attained in that particular area, a new invitation is sent out (in the case of Pamplona, to everyone).

Results

The mammography programme began on 5th March, 1990, with only one unit working during the first 4 months to make sure that all the arrangements had been set up correctly. Although final figures cannot be presented until the first round has been completed, the following data can be considered as advance figures corresponding to the first year. Up to 31st August, 31, 466 invitations to attend had been sent out of which 1,308 have been identified as incorrect due to a number of reasons (see Table 1). From the total figure of 30,158 valid invitations, 25,468 women attended, representing a compliance of

Table 1. Participation

No. of citations	31,466
Reasons for rejection	1,308
- unknown address	702
- disability	61
- mastectomies already performed	271
- pending	274
No. of valid citations	30,158
No. of participants	25,468
Compliance	84.45%

84.45%; a figure which exceeds the anticipated aim and, naturally, the minimum level required for the programme to be effective.

Average compliance in Pamplona, the capital of Navarra, was 83.06%, although it varied from suburb to suburb. Only 75% was reached in the Old Part, the lowest figures for the city. The average age of the population of this part of the city is high; it is not highly structured socially and there are considerable differences in socio-economic terms. The highest compliance (87.46%) was seen in a well-organised lower-middle class suburb, where the health centre and the Women's Association played a major role in "recruitment".

There was a compliance of over 85% in all the areas around Pamplona.

As far as the rural areas are concerned (covered by the mobile unit), the high level of general compliance is noteworthy, over 90% in some areas. Only the northern (mountainous) area shows a lower level of participation, especially the Basque-speaking areas, although until this has been analysed, the phenomenon cannot be attributed to socio-economic factors specific to this area (see Table 2).

Compliance by age group is quite homogeneous, dropping only in the 60-65 age group; this accords well with many other programmes (see Table 3).

Table 2. Participation by area

Area	Total of citations	Justified rejects	Participants	Participation
Permanent unit	17,296	870	13,727	83,57
Pamplona	14,248	709	11,245	83.06
Surrounding area	3,048	161	2,482	85.97
Mobile unit	14,170	438	11,741	85.50
Mountain area	3,676	115	2,795	78.49
Rest of rural area	10,496	363	8,946	87.96

Table 3. Participation by age

Age	Total of citations	Justified rejects	Participants	Participation
< 45 - > 65	-	-	104	-
45 - 49	7,545	299	6,213	85.74
50 - 54	6,563	252	5,451	86.37
55 - 59	7,786	302	6,392	85.41
60-65	9,468	455	7,308	81.08

Conclusion

Breast cancer can be cured. This is the idea that should motivate any campaign of early detection of breast cancer and that should be transmitted, on the one hand, to the population to be screened, i.e., every woman involved, and on the other, to the public health authorities, with the aim of significantly reducing mortality.
Bearing in mind these objectives, high compliance figures become an essential requirement for screening programmes.

REFERENCES

1   Hakama M: Screening. Oxford Text Book of Public Health 1991 (3):91-106
2   Morgan M: Sociological investigations. Oxford Text Book of Public Health 1991 (2):309-329
3   García M: El análisis de la realidad social. Alianza Universidad Textos 1989 pp 489-501
4   Hobs P, Smith A, George MW and Sellwood RA: Acceptors and rejectors of an invitation to undergo breast screening compared with those who referred themselves. J Epidem Commun Health 1980 (34):19-22
5   Eardley A and Elkind A: A pilot study of attendance for breast cancer screening. Soc Sci Med 1990 (30):693-699
6   Puska P, Koskela K, McAlister A et al: Use of lay leaders to promote diffusion of health innovations in a community program: Lessons learned from the North Karelia project. Bulletin of the World Health Organization 1986 (64):437-446
7   Farkuhar JW, Fortmann SP, Flora JA and Macoby N: Methods of communication to influence behaviour. Oxford Text Book of Public Health 1991 (2):331-344
8   Mayer JA and Kellog MC: Promoting mammography appointment making. J Behavioral Med (12):605-611

Breast Cancer Screening in Montpellier

Jean-Louis Lamarque, Jeanine Cherif Cheikh, Joseph Pujol, Patrick Boulet, Jean-Claude Laurent and Jean-Pierre Daures

Département d'Imagerie Médicale, Hôpital Lapeyronie, 555 Route de Ganges, 34059 Montpellier Cedex, France

Experiments conducted over a period of more than 15 years in the United States and in Northern Europe (Great Britain, Holland) have shown that it is possible to reduce mortality rates by 30 to 45% through screening with mammography.

The Montpellier experiment began in June 1990 and is based upon a system still unique in France, consisting of centralised mobile units and presenting the following characteristics.

Organised Mass Screening

It is an example of mass screening in perfect harmony with the principles stated by the World Health Organization in 1968.

The target population are women between the ages of 40 and 70. The test includes 2 angles of incidence per breast and is repeated every 2 years. All women in the target population receive a personal invitation to come to the mobile unit.

Women arrive in the truck and present their invitation at the reception desk. They give the name of the doctor to whom the test results should be sent, whether the test is positive or negative. The examination is carried out by specially trained breast imagery technicians in the absence of doctors. The women then leave and are reminded that in case of a positive test result, they should consult their own doctor.

The planned interview is always reassuring and confidential, the personnal being carefully trained in this field.

Mobile Units

A mobile unit system has been adopted because it is easy to move around, goes out to the women, is more encouraging and makes quality control easier.

The itinerary of the mobile unit is organised by the screening centre according to a map and a chronology, taking into account the geographic distribution of the target population. The arrival of the unit is preceded by several preparatory meetings, attended by doctors from the sector, paramedical personnel, local government officials concerned with health and welfare, a member of the Medical Committee (see below), as well as representatives of various socio-cultural associations. These meetings are open to all interested women: after having been informed about the techniques used for the test, the women may ask questions concerning the screening.

The mobile unit parks according to a calendar established by the screening centre. The centre confers on the location of the unit with the local committees (local imperatives, access facilities, exemplary and incitement value of the location).

All the organisations interested in the screening will be informed of the locations and the dates on which the mobile unit will be on site.

Women between the ages of 40 and 70, who have not received an invitation through official channels, can present themselves voluntarily for screening (a free telephone is at their disposal).

Centralisation

One single centre (the Montpellier Institute for Medico-Biological Imaging: IMIM) takes care of computer management, invitations, analysis and follow-up of the tests. This is also a very important point when setting up quality control.

Second Reading

Second reading is carried out by breast radiology specialists, regularly trained and controlled (both teachers and students).

Rapidity of Test Results

The test results are sent to the woman and her doctor two days after the test. Every evening the tests carried out during the day are returned to the centre at the IMIM. The X-rays are given a second reading by specialists trained in mammographic screening.

About 7% of all tests are considered positive, i.e., they present an anomaly which requires diagnostic control. The woman's name is never known to the doctor performing the reading; anonymity is assured in the form of a number. The central secretariat, which receives the test requiring diagnostic control, sends a letter to the woman informing her that her test presents an anomaly and that it should be examined further. The choice of the diagnostic service is made by the woman and her doctor.

The doctor receives from the central secretariat a letter informing him that the test is positive and that he must decide upon the diagnostic orientation. He should send back the results of the diagnosis and follow-up for a proper evaluation of the screening process.

In the case of a negative test, the woman and her doctor receive a letter saying that the woman will be contacted 2 years later. During this interval, the woman is advised to practise self-examination and to remain under the surveillance of her own doctor or a specialist.

Control of the Results

The medical committee includes a team of epidemiologists which ensures the evalution of the campaign.

Creation of Medical and Female Committees

These committees play a role in the distribution of information and in raising the sensibility to the public. They aim at active support of the medical community and at a maximum level of participation (see Appendix).

The Important Role of the General Practitioner

He is responsible for sending and investigating the results, and should take action in the case of a positive result.

Financing

The test is offered free of charge to women of the District of Montpellier (a grouping of Montpellier and 14 communities around the city) by private and public organisations.

Quality Control

Quality control in organised mass screening is not limited to quality control of the image. It involves a chain in which each link is essential in order to obtain a significant reduction in mortality. The methods of quality control are detailed elsewhere in this monograph.

The First Results from Montpellier

Since 12th November, 1991, 10,937 women

have been screened. The first epidemiological study carried out by Professor J.P. Daures dealt with 5,098 women screened by 8th March, 1991.

The mean participation rate was 64% at the first invitation (participation varying between 59.16% and 74%). There were 396 positive tests (7.76%) in which 30 cancers were discovered. This figure is twice as high as the number of cancers discovered during the same period outside of the screening. Among these cancers, 72.4% were smaller than 1 cm, 27 cancers with negative lymph nodes, 3 with positive lymph nodes and 3 refusals of surgery after biopsy were recorded.

The distribution of the 396 positive tests throughout the structures for diagnosis and treatment is as follows: a) 92.29% in public hospitals, b) 90.7% in private institutions (Centre Recherche et Lutte du Cancer: 24.53%, private practices and clinics: 66.17%).

Conclusion

Although Montpellier is the most medically-minded city in France, the participation rate was about 60% at the first invitation, showing that regular breast surveillance outside screening programmes only reached a small percentage of the population. Thanks to the screening, the percentage of women regularly undergoing breast examination increased from approximately 20% to 80%. It has become evident that this campaign has to be extended to cover the entire department of Hérault. A second mobile unit is in operation since December, 1991, and a third unit will provide screening for the entire department of Hérault every 2 years (between 100,000 and 250,000 women).

Appendix

The Women's Committee for Breast Cancer Screening (C.F.D.C.S.), which was set up in February 1989, is unique in the world. It consists of voluntary female workers, not doctors, and is organised as an association under the law of 1901 (non-profit making) and sponsored by H.R.H. Princess Caroline of Monaco who is taking part in the Hérault Breast Cancer Screening Campaign.

In France, only 20% of women between the ages of 40 and 70 have ever had a mammography. Of the same group it is estimated that only 6% to 8% have mammographs every 2 years. All those regularly undergoing mammography come from the upper socio-professional and cultural strata, a milieu which has access to information.

The aim of the Women's Committee is to ensure that at least 80% of all women in this age group participate in the screening campaigns. The role of the Committee is to provide information so as to increase awareness of the problem, and, during the campaign, to give support to women being screened.

The Women's Committee acts as the contact between the public and the doctors organising the screening. The female volunteers become the special confidants of the women being screened: it is easier to say certain things to members of the Women's Committee than to a doctor, to ask questions that would be embarrassing otherwise ("Is a mammography painful? Dangerous? How long does it take? Is it really free of charge? When will the results be available? Does a positive result mean I have cancer? Etc...").

The Committee has a specially adapted motor-vehicle, the INFOMOBILE, which precedes the MAMMOBILE by a couple of weeks in its tour through the different parts of Montpellier and the communes and villages of the Department. This vehicle circulates throughout the area, and just by displaying the Campaign advertising it encourages women to be tested. It also acts as an office where women can come and ask questions, where they can listen to the arguments and be convinced of the importance of being screened.

Every day some 50 women (of the 400 who are members of the Committee) take an active part in the campaign, distributing leaflets, posters, and documentary information to the public, to local shopkeepers, to doctors, and to para-medical professionals.

The Women's Committee, in conjunction with the Hérault Medical Committee for Breast Cancer Screening, organises open meetings in local community halls, for associations, companies, etc., and provides as much in formation to the public as possible.

It collaborates with the communication department in providing both written and audio-visual information. It takes part in media events publicising the usefulness of the campaign and participates in public gatherings such as fairs, congresses and exhibitions. The Women's Committee telephone service receives around 30 calls a day.

Lastly, through the organising committee, it takes an active part in the planning of the screening sessions.

The 400 members of the Association, created under the 1901 law, elect a Management Board for 4 years. The Management Board in turn elects a Management Committee for 1 year and is composed of 1 president, 2 vice-presidents, 1 general secretary, 1 assistant secretary, 1 treasurer, 1 assistant treasurer.

The Montpellier Institute for Medico-Biological Imaging (I.M.I.M.) provides an office for the Women's Committee with a full time secretary. She runs the freephone service with the help of the voluntary workers.

The Management Committee handles the day-to-day administration and allocates the work to be done according to an "action calendar" closely linked to that of the breast screening organisation.

The women are split up into teams, who take turns in carrying out the Association's activities in the areas to be visited by the Mammobile.

In most of the "medical" towns of France, Paris excepted (1 doctor per 149 inhabitants), the results of the first 5,000 women screened show that 64% turned up for their first appointment, a rate of participation unequalled elsewhere in France.

When compared with traditional methods of diagnosis covering the same geographical area and taken over a comparable period, the screening has enabled twice as many cancers to be traced. This is in large part due to the action of the Women's Committee.

The Bas-Rhin Model: A Non-Centralised Screening Programme

Béatrice Gairard, Robert Renaud, Paul Schaffer and Catherine Guldenfels

ADEMAS, 10 Rue Leicester, 67000 Strasbourg, France

An important issue facing us in France at the moment is to find out the best way to set up an effective national screening system. Can we do this by simply copying the existing models in other countries or is it preferable to envisage different possibilities? *A priori* it proves impossible to copy the existing models as they stand. They are in most instances studies or trials rather than national mass programmes. Furthermore, a certain number of problems specific to our country have to be borne in mind; a degree of individual screening by the private-practice radiologists which is already quite high (1,200,000 mammograms were carried out in asymptomatic women in 1988); a large number of mammographs (2,000 units); the lack of updated, reliable and exhaustive population registers; the fact that it would be impossible to make use of them even if they did exist because of the extremely strict rules laid down by the National Commission on Data Processing and Freedom (Commission Nationale Informatique et Liberté) concerning computerised lists, and the lack of conviction on the part of the GPs who do not encourage the women to participate. This was why, 4 years ago, we proposed and set up a pilot campaign (ADEMAS) in the department of the Bas-Rhin, under the aegis of Europe Against Cancer. The original features of our pilot project are:
- to use the existing structures, i.e. the existing radiology units, both private and public, rather than creating new structures;
- not to use population registers and invitation systems which give rise to many problems, particularly with regard to their quality, completeness and updating;
- fo fit in neatly with the health-care structures, taking into account our code of ethics and our health-care system [1-3].

Many specialists in other countries, although extremely interested in the advantages of this approach, which is unique for the moment, are still sceptical, if not sometimes downright hostile as to its chances of success, claiming that a mass screening operation can only be envisaged if implemented on the basis of population registers and carried out in highly specialised centres which also perform diagnosis and treatment. This is why one of our main objectives is to prove the effectiveness of our system. In order to achieve this, it has been essential to set up a rigorous, high-quality evaluation system, especially since the majority of the radiologists are not specialised in mammography, let alone screening mammography.

Organisation of the Evaluation

Even in the decentralised systems it is essential to set up a coordinating centre which carries out a continuous monitoring of the screening campaign. This monitoring is based on a system of registration and management of data which can be used for cross-referencing the successive data concerning the screening of the same individual in the target population as well as the results of diagnosis and treatment, should they be required. The necessary prerequisites for such a continuous monitoring system are:

- knowledge of the structure of the target population and the changes in this population over time;
- a register, with names, of all the women screened and, for the positives, the input of the diagnostic and treatment results;
- a cancer register, which makes it possible to be aware of the interval cancers and the "false negatives" (missed cancers);
- comparisons of the deaths in the target population as compared with the non-screened women in order to evaluate specific mortality;
- knowledge of what happens before, in parallel with and outside of the screening campaign among the female population of the Bas-Rhin department.

Participation of the Target Population

The programme evaluates the eligibility of the women and their compliance. In the example of the department of the Bas-Rhin, the women are not invited to attend individually and personally; although the screening is free of charge, no voucher is sent out beforehand. Any woman who wishes to undergo a screening examination may either present herself directly or may be referred by her doctor to the radiologist of her choice as long as he is on the list of radiologists authorised by the coordinating centre and the Social Security systems.

To date, the participation of women is not lower than that of other French programmes using personalised invitations. As in other European countries, there is in all cases a slightly higher participation in rural than in urban areas.

Further studies of women's motivation, and particularly an investigation of the role of the referring doctor, such as the GP, should therefore be undertaken. It is necessary to evaluate the number of diagnostic mammograms and systematic examinations undertaken outside the screening: this procedure has been performed for 5 to 10% of the women during the first year.

Evaluation of the Referring Doctors

Many of the GPs are not familiar with the re-

quirements of a screening programme and find it difficult to distinguish between a screening test and diagnostic examination. This lack of scientific knowledge is often upheld by the contradictory articles which regularly appear in the medical press and by the fallacious arguments of the radiologists who have refused to participate in the programme. This is why some of them are reluctant to apply to their own patients the rules of a public health programme and, in the final analysis, they deprive them of the benefits of an organised screening. We frequently have the impression that our message has not been properly received and that we should do a great deal more to provide information and training for the medical practitioners.

The participation of gynaecologists is, on the whole, relatively good. We observe that it is the gynaecologist who has encouraged the women to attend, or is the person whom 53% of the women participating in the screening wish to receive their results from. By contrast, out of all the GPs nominated, only 40% were chosen and this by only 5 women or fewer as the person to pass on to them the results of the screening [3].

It is interesting to compare these results with those of Spain (European Pilot Programme of Navarra) where the high participation rate (85% of the population) seems to be attributable to the very active role of the family doctor who may encourage his patients to participate [4]. In France, such behaviour is contrary to the rules concerning the free choice of a doctor, even though similar experiments are now being attempted within the specific framework of public health action.

Evaluation of the Results of the Screening Mammograms

This evaluation requires the establishment of a cancer register as well as the drawing up of lists of all the cytological and histological mammary examinations. In this way, we are able to measure the changes in incidence, in the stage at the time of diagnosis of incident cancers, as well as improvement in their treatment, sensitivity, specificity, and positive predictive value.

Evaluation of the Structures and Set Up

The Radiologists

In the majority of the French departments where a system of this kind has been established, most of the radiologists participate in the screening. However, it is quite certain that the number of screening mammograms carried out annually varies greatly. This being the case, one might be afraid of heterogeneous results in the reading of the mammograms as well as a lack of training among the readers due to the large numbers involved.

In order to obtain a homogeneous and satisfactory result, the radiologist who has carried out the mammogram checks its quality and sends it, together with his interpretation, to the coordinating centre. A second reading is carried out by radiologists who are specialised in mammography and, in a case of disagreement, a third reading is carried out by a third reader in the presence of the other two. In this way the third reading also provides in-service training for all the readers.

Analysis of the first results of the interpretation of the mammograms carried out within the Bas-Rhin experiment has shown that at the first reading 9.5% of the mammograms were considered positive. At the second reading, carried out by a specialised radiologist, the percentage of positives dropped to 7.7 and remained so after the third reading. If one relates the results of the first and second readings to the results of the diagnostic examinations and to the histological results, it is noticeable that for the mammograms which had been considered positive at the first reading, but negative at the second and third, few cancers had been discovered, whereas for those mammograms considered negative by the first reader and positive by the other two, a certain number of cancers have been diagnosed and their number represents roughly one-fifth of the cancers. These results indicate the importance of a second reading for all the mammograms and not only for the positive results of the first reading.

The heterogeneous nature of the experience of the different radiologists and the difficulties in training those with little practical experience lead us to question the exact role played by the non-specialised radiologists in a national screening programme. Will we continue to need a second reading by radiologists specialised in breast imaging, thus considerably reducing the role and responsibility of the non-specialists, or will they be capable of carrying out this screening without a second reading? Should this second reading be restricted to those mammograms alone which were positive at the first reading as is the case for the other pilot projects in France, or should it be carried out for all mammograms regardless of the result of the first reading? Who should carry out the second reading? Should it be a specialist in mammography or another radiologist without specialist training? Quite apart from the psychological aspects of this last solution, it must be pointed out that the second reading carried out by non-specialists involves the risk of a considerable increase in the number of false positives without any decrease in the number of false negatives.

Quality Assurance of the Screening Procedure

It is essential that any initiative taken in a given region be backed up by a protocol of quality assurance which must be scrupulously complied with by all the participants in the campaign.

Due to the large number of examinations carried out, it is indeed absolutely necessary to guarantee the non-deterioration of the minimum technical performance of the material, to ensure that the results obtained using different equipment can be easily compared and to continue to try to improve the quality of the radiographic image whilst keeping the radiation level of the patients as low as possible.

It is desirable that the different stages of a protocol on quality control should be carried out by a body independent of the coordination centre, as well as of the firms providing the material. The protocol on quality assurance must cover the 4 different links in the radiological chain: the production, reception, processing and viewing of the image. The setting up of such a system of quality assurance can only be successful if the different partners, i.e. the radiologists and manufacturers, collaborate in a fruitful and construc-

tive way. The objectives to be achieved are the following:
- improving the quality of the image and maintaining it at its optimal position;
- reducing the radiation dose to the lowest possible level;
- improving the collective reproducibility of the different views.

This last point is particularly important in a decentralised system so as to ensure that the readers do not have to interpret mammograms carried out in very different conditions.

Evaluation of the Diagnostic Procedures

In a good screening programme, the diagnostic procedures must be of as high a quality as the screening examinations. However, in most of the experimental sites in France, the quality control of these diagnostic procedures is not in the hands of the organisers since, once the test has been carried out and the result communicated, the patient's doctor and the radiologist who carry out these procedures are then free to decide how to proceed. This is why it seems important to us that the evaluation of the diagnostic procedures should be carried out by investigating the numbers of positive results, the result of the biopsies carried out (where the results are nominal), and by the number of interval cancers. Some of the difficulties encountered in providing quality control of these procedures arise from the fact that these women have the possibility of going for a second or third opinion to other radiologists who may have differing opinions as to the possible indication for a biopsy. Furthermore, the less experienced radiologists tend to request another check in the interim period between screening rounds, which also affects the quality of the procedure.

Evaluation of Needle Biopsy and Pathological Examination

All members of a group of pathologists within a programme must agree to standardise their reports. In order to do so, it is desirable that they fill out a standardised form which sets out all the information required by the coordi-

nating centre. In the Bas-Rhin, they have agreed to complete these forms for all the needle biopsies and the biopsies performed for all the women of the department. In this way, it is possible to follow up all cases and to compare cytological and pathological data to provide the quality control of the whole programme.

It is equally necessary to carry out the training for all the pathologists, and evaluation and training meetings organised by those in charge of the programmes and who already have considerable experience may take place.

Evaluation of the Surgical Treatment

In decentralised systems, any surgery carried out as a result of anomalies discovered following a screening may also be undertaken within the existing oncological or gynaecological surgical services of the department. This being the case, at this stage too we find different treatment methods used amongst the surgeons. As for the pathologists, it is possible to envisage ongoing training courses. But it is thanks to the results of the follow-up of patients and the comparison of information about treatment methods that it will be possible to provide useful information about the treatment of the cancers detected. It must be added that treatment protocols must be further studied in the treatment of certain lesions such as early cancers, in situ cancers and borderline lesions.

Conclusions

Screening programmes for breast cancer based on private practice structures have been organised in the Department of the Bas-Rhin by ADEMAS. The purpose of such programmes is to define the practical requirements needed to screen for this cancer given these special characteristics. The first results justify our thinking that the factors we have selected should allow for breast cancer screening with a participation rate which may be as high as 60%, at an acceptable cost in countries with a health system similar to that in France. We have reason to believe that the mammograms can be properly carried out, with a good quality interpretation, as long as a second reading is performed by specialised radiologists and the diagnosis and treatment are also satisfactory. The best conditions in which to obtain a sufficiently high degree of participation of the women, the cooperation of the referring doctors and in particular that of the gynaecologists and the GPs, still remain to be defined. Information and awareness campaigns for the medical practitioners are required and proper training for the radiologists carrying out the mammograms must be provided. At the moment it is still necessary to have a second reading by the specialised radiologists for all the screening mammograms. Finally, a quality-assurance system must be envisaged for all the stages in the procedure, covering the screening proper as well as diagnosis and treatment.

REFERENCES

1   Renaud R, Gairard B, Schaffer P, Haehnel P, Dale G: Définition et principes du dépistage du cancer du sein. In: Lansac J, Lefloch O, Bougnoux Ph (eds) Dépistage du Cancer du Sein et Conséquences Thérapeutiques. Masson, Paris 1989 pp 1-14

2   Renaud R, Schaffer P, Gairard B, Haehnel P, Dale G, Wahl P, Methlin G, Irrmann M, Lion J, Charton B: La campagne pilote européenne de dépistage du cancer du sein dans le Bas-Rhin. In: Lansac J, Lefloch O, Bougnoux Ph (eds) Dépistage du Cancer du Sein et Conséquences Thérapeutiques. Masson, Paris 1989 pp 29-42

3   Renaud R, Schaffer P, Gairard B, Dale G, Haehnel P, Kleitz C, Guldenfels C: Principes et premiers résultats de la campagne européenne de dépistage du cancer du sein dans le Bas-Rhin. Bull Acad Natle Méd 1991 (175,1):129-147

4   Réunion des experts de l'Europe Contre le Cancer, sous-comité dépistage du cancer du sein. Vougliameni, Greece, September 1991

Non-Invasive Breast Cancer: An Important Screening Problem

Ingvar Andersson [1] and Debra M. Ikeda [2]

1   Department of Radiology, Malmö General Hospital, 21401 Malmö, Sweden
2   Department of Radiology, Stanford University Medical Center, 300 Pasteur Drive, Stanford, CA 94304, USA

In the past, breast carcinoma *in situ* (CIS) comprised only a small percentage of all breast cancers and the traditional treatment, mastectomy, resulted in close to 100% cure [1-4]. During the last 2 decades, the scenario has changed: due to the widespread use of mammography many more *in situ* carcinomas are detected, comprising up to 20% of cancers in screening-detected series [5-8]. Simultaneously, there has been a trend towards breast conserving surgery [9-11]. This has raised important questions about the natural history of the disease; does CIS always proceed to invasive carcinoma? If not, are there accurate prognostic indicators to determine which CIS are more aggressive? What is the prevalence of multifocal disease, how is it assessed, and what is its clinical significance? What is the optimal extent of surgery for CIS? What is the effect of radiation therapy? Can progression to invasive disease be prevented by medication?

Some studies suggest that CIS starts as benign epithelial proliferation, progressing through increasing degrees of atypia to intraductal (DCIS) or intralobular (LCIS) carcinoma and finally to invasive carcinoma [12, 13].

The mammographic detection of DCIS is most commonly due to the occurrence of calcifications (often called microcalcifications) in the involved mammary duct. Similar calcifications are sometimes seen in atypical epithelial hyperplasia [14]. Thus, if atypical hyperplasia progresses to CIS and CIS progresses to invasive cancer, mammography has the potential to play a significant role in preventing development of invasive carcinoma from such lesions. On the other hand, LCIS practi-cally never produces pathologic mammographic changes.

The large number of mammographically-detected cases of DCIS in recent years has created new problems and raised questions: does DCIS detected by mammography act in the same biological manner as DCIS detected clinically? What proportion of mammographically-detected DCIS is biologically significant? Can this proportion be identified?

Histology

Traditionally, 2 types of CIS have been defined, ductal (DCIS) and lobular (LCIS) [12,15]. Both are believed to originate in the terminal ductular lobular units of the breasts [16]. In both types the malignant epithelial cells are confined to the lumina of the ducts or lobules without penetration of the basement membrane as seen by light microscopy. In DCIS there may or may not be reactive stromal changes such as fibrosis, elastosis and inflammatory reaction surrounding the involved ducts and lobules.

DCIS exhibits various growth patterns: solid, cribriform, papillary, and micropapillary with or without so-called comedo-necrosis [17]. The term "comedo" (meaning worm) refers to the gross appearance of comedo-like structures protruding from breast ducts on the cut surface of a pathological specimen containing this type of DCIS. This represents a coagulation necrosis of epithelial cells and is most often seen with a solid growth pattern. Subsequently, the necrotic core may undergo dystrophic calcification. The resulting calcifications form the basis for radiographic detection of most cases of DCIS [18,19].

The cellular atypia is usually more severe in the comedo-type carcinomas than in the micropapillary or cribriform types. The comedo-type DCIS is usually considered to have a greater potential for invasion and therefore a graver prognosis [20,21].

Some pathologists classify DCIS into 2 main categories: 1) "classical" comedo carcinoma, characterised by large cells with atypical nuclei and the presence of necrotic material in the ducts, and 2) cribriform and micropapillary CIS. In most cases a mixture of various types is seen, albeit with one dominant type.

Another classification of DCIS by tumour growth patterns has been presented by Andersen et al. [22]: 1) *microfocal* growth pattern involving one or a few lobules or ducts, usually smaller than 1 mm but sometimes 3 to 5 mm in diameter without stromal reaction; 2) *diffuse* growth pattern involving normally distributed ducts, the involvement can be focal or extensive and stromal fibrosis and inflammatory reaction are often observed; 3) *tumour-forming* growth pattern characterised by densely packed glandular structures with stromal fibrosis and inflammatory changes.

As mentioned above, the existence of a continuum from epithelial hyperplasia, through atypical epithelial changes to frank CIS has been suggested by several authors [12,13]. The relative risk to develop an invasive carcinoma has been calculated for women with a surgical biopsy showing moderate florid hyperplasia versus age-matched healthy women to be 1.5 to 2.0. Women with atypical ductal (ADH) or lobular hyperplasia have a relative risk of 4 to 5. The relative risk of developing an invasive carcinoma would be 8 to 10 with both ADH and a first-degree relative with a history of breast cancer [23-25]. However, the distinction between severe ADH and CIS is difficult, with substantial interobserver variation even among expert pathologists [26].

By definition, CIS does not penetrate the basement membrane, which in practice may sometimes be difficult to assess. If CIS is extensive, the risk of sampling error increases. For these and other reasons invasive cancer may be missed, probably accounting for axillary metastases seen in a few percent of

DCIS cases and also for breast cancer mortality in an even smaller proportion of patients [27,28]. The occurrence of microscopic foci of invasion has been found to correlate with histologic subtype, being more common with the comedo-type of CIS [20], and with the extent of DCIS. Lagios et al. found occult invasion in 50% of breasts with DCIS 55 mm in extent or larger and in none of 60 patients with DCIS 25 mm or smaller [29]. Two of 55 patients (3.6%) with DCIS of a median extent of 50 mm had axillary micrometastases.

Multifocality - Multicentricity

Multifocality usually refers to the presence of multiple foci of CIS in the same quadrant while multicentricity refers to foci in different quadrants. However, the definition of these terms varies and they are often used interchangeably. For purposes of this discussion, the term multifocal will be used as a description of separate foci of disease, with normal tissue in between these foci. A large number of studies show that DCIS is often multifocal. The data on this frequency varies, probably due to differences in the extent of sampling. In one study, 19 of 33 patients (58%) who had an excisional biopsy for DCIS, who then underwent subcutaneous mastectomy, had additional foci of DCIS in the mastectomy specimens [30]. Rosen et al. reported residual non-invasive carcinoma in 60% of mastectomy specimens after biopsy for DCIS, with 33% outside the original quadrant biopsied [31].

Similar findings have been reported by others [32-34]. Ciatto found multifocality of DCIS in 76% (71 of 93) of the cases [35]. In an autopsy series of 20- to 54-year-old women, foci of DCIS were found in more than one quadrant in 7 out of 15 cases [36]. Holland et al. differ from most others and found that DCIS almost always involves only one region of the breast, with contiguous growth of DCIS within ducts of that region [37]. However, most lesions in the series of Holland et al. were large, with about a quarter extending over more than one quadrant.

Lagios et al. found that the frequency of multifocality correlated with the size of the tumour

[38]. They found 13 of 24 lesions larger than 25 mm were multifocal, compared to 4 of 24 smaller lesions. In conclusion, it is apparent that DCIS often consists of several separate foci, most of which are located in the same quadrant but some in other quadrants.

Bilaterality

DCIS has been shown to carry an increased risk of contralateral breast cancer, although less than LCIS. DCIS was shown to be bilateral in 7 of 36 cases (19%) in a series of patients undergoing contralateral subcutaneous mastectomy after ipsilateral diagnosis of DCIS [30]. In another series, 7 of 132 women (5%) with DCIS followed for a median of 7 years developed contralateral breast carcinoma (4 invasive, 2 DCIS, 1 LCIS) [39].
In a Danish autopsy series of 110 young and middle-aged women, 5 of 15 cases of DCIS found at autopsy were bilateral [36].
Ciatto et al. reported contralateral breast cancer (invasive and non-invasive) in a total of 23 of 156 patients (15%), 9 of whom had been diagnosed with cancer before the discovery of DCIS in the other breast [35].

Incidence and Age Distribution

Data on the incidence and age distribution of DCIS varies substantially in the literature, mainly due to the extent in which mammography was used for diagnosis and screening.
In the city of Malmö, 132 patients were diagnosed with DCIS out of a total of 1,693 breast cancer cases over a 9-year period (1976-1984) during which half of the population aged 45 to 69 years was invited to screening with mammography; mammography was also available for symptomatic patients [39]. The incidence of DCIS was 14.9 per 100,000 woman years with a trend towards the highest incidence of DCIS among middle-aged (45-60 years old) women. Seventy-five percent of the patients had a positive mammogram and in 46% mammography was the only modality indicating carcinoma.

Sunshine et al. also found CIS (mostly DCIS) to be more common among pre- and peri-menopausal women as compared to post-menopausal women [3]. Their material consisted mainly of symptomatic patients. A similar trend in age distribution was found by Ciatto et al. [35].
Two Danish autopsy studies with meticulous sampling of the breasts showed DCIS in 11 of 77 (14%) and in 15 of 109 (14%) patients without previously known breast cancer [36,40]. This is a much higher prevalence than the cumulated risk of being diagnosed with CIS in a corresponding Danish population not subjected to breast cancer screening with mammography (less than 1% between ages 20 and 75). It was concluded that at most one-third of all *in situ* lesions progress to clinically invasive breast cancer [41].

Treatment

DCIS presents a therapeutic dilemma. The trend towards breast conserving surgery for invasive carcinoma makes it seem illogical to treat DCIS more aggressively, i.e., with mastectomy. On the other hand, it was reported that patients undergoing only excisional biopsy for what was believed to be benign disease but which was retrospectively diagnosed as DCIS had a cancer recurrence rate of about 25% [28,42,43]. Most recurrences were invasive and occurred in the same quadrant as the initial biopsy. About 10% of the patients in each series died of breast cancer during the period of follow-up. These early studies included mostly patients with non-comedo type DCIS. However, similar results have been reported in later series [4].
Lagios et al. found "occult" invasion in mastectomy specimens after excisional biopsy for DCIS in approximately 50% of patients with DCIS with an extension of more than 45 mm, and in none less than 45 mm, provided that the initial excision had been adequate [29]. In a series of 79 patients with mostly mammographically-detected DCIS lesions (measuring 25 mm or less) treated with "tylectomy" without radiation, 8 patients (10%) recurred (4 invasive, 4 non-invasive) in the immediate vicinity of the original site [29]. Recurrence

was strongly related to high-grade nuclear morphology and comedo-necrosis in the initial lesion. The follow-up period in this series was 48 months (median 44 months). Silverstein et al. reported similar results, although their inclusion criteria were somewhat different [44].

Bornstein et al. [46] pointed out the importance of careful mammographic and pathologic assessment to reduce the local recurrence rate.

Recurrences may be related to multifocal (multicentric), non-invasive disease developing into invasive disease, or to the presence of occult, microinvasive disease at the time of initial surgery. The addition of postoperative radiation seems to reduce the recurrence rate [4,45,46].

Comparison of published data regarding the effect of different treatments is impeded by the differences in the inclusion criteria in the various studies and how these criteria are assessed. Randomised studies are ongoing comparing the effect of local excision with and without radiation and with and without tamoxifen.

In summary, the optimum treatment for DCIS remains to be defined and should possibly be varied, depending upon biological activity. Prognostic parameters for DCIS need to be assessed. Currently, the extent of the disease, nuclear grade and the presence of comedo necrosis seem to be important. Thymidine labelling index, DNA ploidy and NEU-protein overexpression may be of additional value [47-49].

Mammography

Mammography plays a key role in the detection of DCIS due to its ability to identify calcifications. However, a proportion of DCIS will present clinically as a breast mass or thickening. Occasionally, DCIS will present clinically with bloody or sudden, copious serous nipple discharge and/or Paget's disease of the nipple.

In an analysis of a consecutive series of DCIS (190 cases), we found that the calcifications were the dominant indicator of malignancy in 62% (117 women) of the cases [50]. The remaining 73 women had either negative mammograms (30 women, 16%) or soft tissue changes other than calcifications (43 women, 22%). The majority of DCIS cases without calcifications had clinical findings, mostly a palpable mass, thickening, bloody discharge or Paget's disease of the nipple.

In a material selected on the basis of needle localisation of non-palpable lesions, the vast majority of patients reported by Dershaw et al. [18] had calcifications on mammography (53 out of 54 cases). Stomper et al. reported a material selected on the basis of similar criteria with only 10% (10 of 100) of the lesions presenting as soft-tissue abnormality [19].

Calcifications in DCIS typically vary in size, form and density with a linear (ductal) or branching arrangement. Calcifications associated with benign disease tend to be rounded with more uniform density. They tend to be either scattered or arranged in groups [51]. Lanyi suggests that the calcification cluster shape may be important. In an analysis of 153 clusters of calcifications in malignancies, he found no round or oval clusters. The most common calcification cluster shape of malignant aetiology was triangular, reflecting the anatomic distribution of breast ducts [52].

Figure 1 shows characteristic calcifications with suspicious linear and branching appearance; they vary in density, shape, and size. Even when the calcifications form casts, the individual calcifications can usually be identified, giving the casts a more or less irregular appearance. This is in contradistinction to so-called plasma cell mastitis where the ductal calcifications are homogenously dense and have a smooth outline. The pattern seen in Figure 1 is virtually pathognomonic of DCIS. Differential diagnoses include atypical ductal hyperplasia and possible calcification of inspissated benign ductal material (Fig. 2).

The type of calcifications seen in Figure 1 is associated with the comedo-type DCIS and represents dystrophic calcification of necrotic material in the core of a solid intraluminal carcinoma growth in dilated ducts. Sometimes the widened ducts can be seen as soft-tissue structures (Fig. 3), either duct-like, nodular or as a diffuse soft-tissue density.

DCIS of cribriform or micropapillary type is occasionally associated with less characteristic calcifications or no calcifications at all

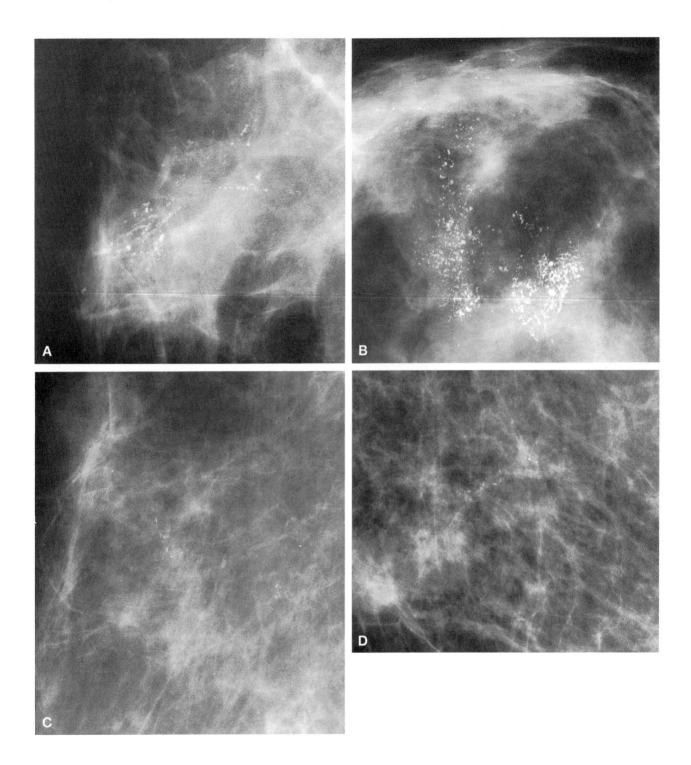

Fig. 1A. Irregular calcifications varying in size, density, and form. A linear (ductal) and branching arrangement is apparent. This pattern is characteristic of DCIS of the comedo type
Fig. 1B. Polymorphic calcifications with a predominantly random distribution in a patient with extensive DCIS. In some areas a ductal arrangement can be seen
Fig. 1C. Magnification view of 2 small clusters of polymorphic calcifications, one of which shows a ductal arrangement. On microscopy, multiple foci of DCIS of the comedo type were found
Fig. 1D. Magnification view showing a limited area of irregular calcifications without definite ductal arrangement. Microscopy showed DCIS with a small focus of invasive disease

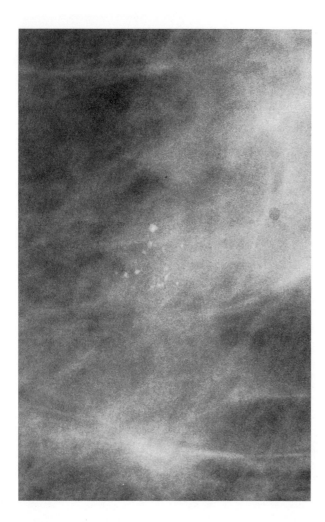

Fig. 2. Magnified view of a 5 mm cluster of polymorphic calcifications. Microscopy showed atypical ductal hyperplasia

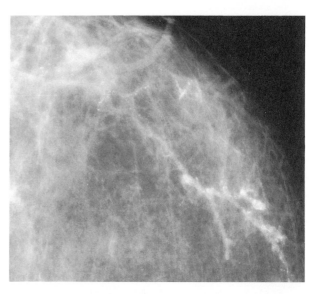

Fig. 3. Screening mammogram shows a dilated duct visible due to soft tissue opacity and calcifications. Microscopy showed DCIS of the comedo type

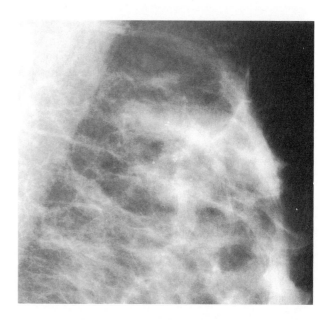

Fig. 4. Asymptomatic woman. Moderate numbers of clustered and scattered calcifications without special characteristics. Microscopy revealed extensive DCIS of predominantly micropapillary type, including and extending far beyond the region of calcifications

(Fig. 4). The pathological basis for these calcifications is different from comedo carcinoma in that the cribriform micropapillary carcinomas have more rounded, psammomatous calcifications which are formed in the lattice created by the intraluminal epithelial growth [52].

In cases like the ones illustrated in Figure 1, microinvasion cannot be excluded radiographically. However, in the absence of a soft-tissue mass one can assume that the carcinoma is going to be predominantly noninvasive.

In general, the 2 main types of breast calcifications which have been identified are calcium phosphate and calcium oxalate [53-55]. Calcium phosphate has mostly been associated with both DCIS and infiltrating carcinoma, while calcium oxalate has been associated with benign disease and LCIS. It is of interest to note that calcium oxalate is not always seen in breast specimens stained with haematoxylin and eosin or with the von Kossa stain [56].

As mentioned earlier, DCIS may present with radiographic patterns other than calcifications. In our series of 190 cases of DCIS, 15 patients had circumscribed masses and 12 had various prominent duct and nodular patterns [50]. Another 16 patients showed still other soft-tissue changes including focal architectural distortion.

Seven of the patients with circumscribed masses represented intracystic cancers, which by definition are considered intraductal (Fig. 5). DCIS other than the intracystic carcinomas may form a more or less well-circumscribed density due to conglomeration of ducts, reactive fibrosis and elastosis.

Asymmetric prominent duct pattern is a relatively common finding and in the majority of cases has no special significance. However, the combination with clinical symptoms, especially bloody or serous discharge, or Paget's disease of the nipple, should alert the radiologist to the possibility of intraductal

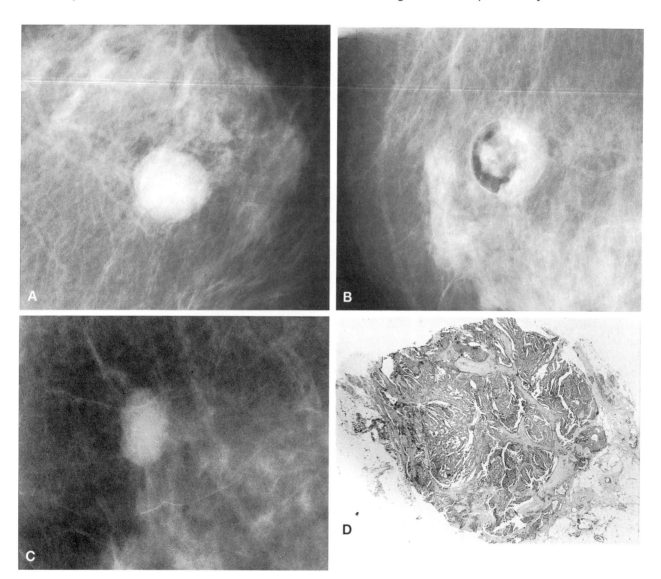

Fig. 5A. Well-marginated, 1.7 cm, dense mass which on aspiration turned out to be cystic with bloody fluid
Fig. 5B. Pneumocystogram shows the mass in 5A to be an intracystic carcinoma outlined by air. On microscopy an intracystic, non-invasive carcinoma was found
Fig. 5C. A 5 x 10 mm, fairly well-circumscribed nodule represents DCIS growing as a solid mass
Fig. 5D. The tumour in 5C consists of intraductal cancerous proliferations (haematoxylin-eosin, 3 times the original magnification)

Reprinted with permission from Radiology [50]

carcinoma (Fig. 6). The presence of DCIS in these cases may be confirmed by galactography and cytology. Figure 7 shows a case with extensive intraductal carcinoma demonstrated by galactography. In this case, calcifications were seen in a small part of the lesion.

Sometimes, DCIS may be diagnosed on the basis of a spiculated lesion or in an area of architectural distortion representing a radial scar. Not uncommonly, epithelial proliferations are seen in the ducts and nodules retracted towards the centre of a radial scar and sometimes even frank DCIS. Sometimes cal-

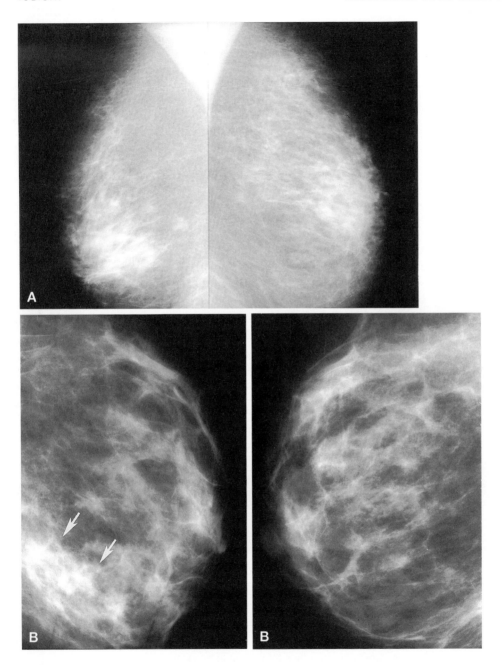

Fig. 6A. Asymmetric prominent duct pattern in the the upper left breast of a woman who had scanty, intermittent bloody discharge. Breast physical examination was normal. Microscopy showed extensive intraductal carcinoma of micropapillary type

Fig. 6B. Asymmetric non-specific density (arrows) in the lower left breast in a patient with Paget's disease of the nipple. Microscopy showed extensive DCIS with Paget's disease of the nipple

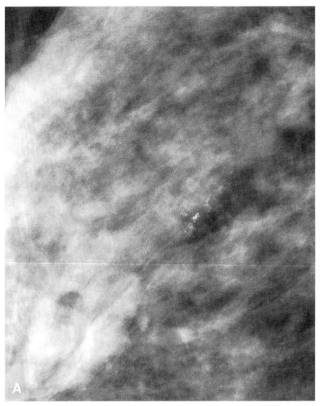
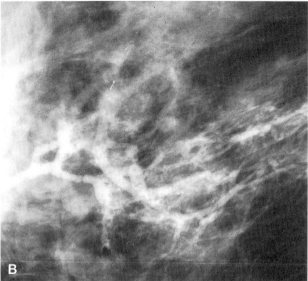

Fig. 7A. Patient with bloody discharge. A small area of clustered, irregular calcifications is seen. Also, note the prominent duct pattern of the parenchyma

Fig. 7B. Galactography showing numerous intraluminal filling defects, over a much more extensive region than suggested by the focus of calcifications. Microscopy showed extensive DCIS in the region of the calcifications and in all quadrants of the breast. Numerous papillomas were also found

cifications are seen on the mammogram around a radial scar.

Paget's disease of the nipple presents clinically as an eczematous lesion on the nipple, sometimes extending onto the areola. Microscopically, there is an invasion of the epidermis by characteristic large, pale Paget cells. This is practically always combined with DCIS in one or several ducts of the nipple. The cancerous lesion may be limited to the nipple or combined with non-invasive or invasive disease elsewhere in the breast.

Extent of DCIS Versus Calcification

On microscopic examination it is very common to find DCIS outside the area of mam-

mographically-visualised calcifications.

Figure 7 shows a case where DCIS was demonstrated by galactography to be far more extensive than suggested by the calcifications. Holland et al. have shown that the magnitude of this discrepancy between the extent of DCIS suggested by mammography and that which is found at biopsy is related to the histologic type of DCIS [37]. In their material, which was dominated by relatively large lesions, 8 of 50 cases of predominantly comedo type showed a discrepancy larger than 20 mm on the pathological specimens compared to the mammographic findings. The corresponding figure for predominantly micropapillary-cribriform DCIS was 15 of 32 cases.

In the medico-legal autopsy study of Nielsen et al., in which the breasts of 110 women were examined histopathologically and with specimen radiography, 9 of 15 cases of DCIS were not visible on specimen radiography.

As a consequence, one would assume that a relatively generous surgical excision is necessary to achieve tumour-free margins around a focus of DCIS.

X-Ray Guided Fine-Needle Aspiration Biopsy

In experienced hands, X-ray guided fine-needle aspiration biopsy represents a valuable technique to further evaluate clusters of calcifications by cytology [57-59]. Calcification localisation can be performed with a stereotactic or coordinate grid technique. With meticulous sampling and correlation of mammographic, cytologic and clinical findings, the number of false-negative results can be kept to a minimum. The advantages to fine-needle biopsy include reduction of the number of unnecessary surgical biopsies and, if given a clear cytologic cancer diagnosis, the surgical procedure can be modified accordingly, i.e., a more extensive excision may be performed to achieve tumour-free breast specimen margins in the first biopsy. One limitation of cytology is the fact that the presence of invasion cannot be determined, and axillary dissection may need to be performed as a second surgical procedure.

The Management of Patients with Calcifications

Breast calcifications are a very common finding at mammography. Some patterns of calcifications are highly characteristic of benign disease, others are characteristic of malignant disease as discussed above. In between these extremes there is a gray zone of calcifications indeterminate for malignancy.

In an attempt to classify calcifications into some simple groups and to assess the probability of carcinoma for these groups, we recommended a surgical biopsy for all clusters containing 5 or more calcifications without obvious mass and not representing obviously benign calcifications such as those seen in plasma cell mastitis, fibroadenomas and arteries [51]. The results of this study are summarised in Table 1. Naturally, the classification of calcifications into various categories is subjective to some extent. This notwithstanding, it seemed clear that it was possible to make rough estimates of the risk of carcinoma for broad categories of calcifications. It should be noted that the 3 cases of LCIS in risk group 1 were considered to be incidental findings in areas adjacent to the areas of calcifications, usually representing fibrocystic disease. It was concluded that recommendation for a surgical biopsy would be appropriate for all risk groups except for risk group 1. For this group, follow-up was considered adequate with a repeat mammogram at 6 and 12 months. Any increase in the number of calcifications should prompt a surgical biopsy unless they are clearly benign, for example, of "teacup" type seen in microcystic disease.

The number of calcifications is less important than the morphology and arrangement of the calcifications. Five calcifications is not a magic number to suggest surgical biopsy upon, even if it is practical to have a threshold level above which biopsy is recommended.

By the same token, the size of a calcification cluster is not as important as the calcification shapes, from a diagnostic point of view.

Table 1. Radiographic appearance of calcifications and risk of malignancy

Risk group	Radiographic characteristis of calc.	Carcinomas N	%
1.	a) rounded b) "cloudy" c) "tea cups"	3/54	6
2.	as in risk group 1 with some irregular calcifications	18/75	24
3.	a) irregular, few b) possible ductal arrangement	24/58	41
4.	a) irregular, abundant b) definitive ductal arrangement	25/26	96

Modified after Sigfusson et al. [51]

Measures to increase imaging resolution to evaluate calcification shapes such as magnification or coned-down views, are important especially in borderline cases [60,61]. In addition, the number of calcifications are seen to greater advantage on magnification views compared to regular views.

Those calcifications which display features of malignancy on such views will proceed to surgical biopsy. Women with calcifications of a clearly benign origin will be returned to mammographic screening. However, some clustered calcifications will be indeterminate for malignancy despite optimal evaluation with magnification views. A portion of these patients will proceed to surgical biopsy due to suspicious clinical findings and/or the inclinations of the patient and her referring physician. However, some calcifications of low suspicion for malignancy may be followed appropriately with short-term mammography and physical examination because of a relatively low predictive value of carcinoma [62,63]. These would include rounded, regular, sharply defined calcifications. The feasibility of implementing radiographic follow-up has been discussed at length [64].

Continuous correlation of radiographic findings with pathology is important as part of a quality-assurance programme to establish a reference base for policies on the management of clustered calcifications [64]. A positive predictive value as low as 10% has been considered acceptable to maximise the number of early carcinomas found in screening programmes by some groups [65]. Others advocate positive predictive values of 40% [66]. However, we agree with Hall et al. that a high specificity and a high predictive value are important in a screening programme. Currently, 3 of 4 surgical procedures in the Malmö mammography screening programme show cancer after a thorough work-up, including X-ray guided fine-needle aspiration.

Summary and Conclusions

DCIS is a heterogenous group of lesions microscopically, radiographically, and with regard to their biologic activity. The comedo type (solid growth pattern with central necrosis and large pleomorphic cells on histology) is usually thought to be of greater biological significance compared to the other *in situ* forms. The prognosis of these lesions may correlate with biological markers such as oncogenes and DNA ploidy.

DCIS is often multifocal but is usually limited to one portion (quadrant) of the breast. It is thought that with increasing size or extent of DCIS the probability of microinvasion increases. The presence of microinvasion cannot be determined on the mammogram.

The microscopic extension of DCIS is often greater than suggested by the calcifications seen on the mammogram. The incidence of DCIS varies with the use of mammography, with more DCIS lesions identified in those programmes which use mammography to a larger extent. Autopsy studies and other data indicate that a proportion of DCIS will never surface clinically. DCIS is usually detected by the presence of calcifications which form within the ducts. Such calcifications have a radiographic spectrum of appearances ranging from a very characteristic irregular branching pattern to calcifications which are non-specific. With experience, a rough estimate of the probability of malignancy represented by such clustered calcifications can be made. X-ray guided fine-needle aspiration biopsy for cytology is valuable in the evaluation and management of patients with clustered calcifications. DCIS may less frequently present radiographically as circumscribed tumours, nodules, or prominent duct pattern.

Continuous correlation between mammographic findings, recommendations for surgical biopsy, and the pathology should be performed in screening centres as a basis for both quality control and guidelines in the management of clustered calcifications detected on mammography.

REFERENCES

1   Schuh ME, Nemoto T, Penetrante RB, Rosner D, Dao TL: Intraductal carcinoma: analysis of presentation, pathologic findings and outcome of disease. Arch Surg 1986 (121):1303-1307

2   Rosner D, Bedwani RN, Vana J, Baker HW, Murphy GP: Non-invasive breast carcinoma: results of a national survey by the American College of Surgeons. Ann Surg 1980 (192):139-147

3   Sunshine JA, Moseley HS, Fletcher WS, Krippaehne WW: Breast carcinoma in situ: a retrospective review of 112 cases with a minimum 10 year follow-up. Am J Surg 1985 (150):44-51

4   Fisher ER, Sass R, Fisher B, Wickerham L, Paik SM: Pathologic findings from the National Surgical Adjuvant Breast Project (protocol 6). I. Intraductal carcinoma (DCIS). Cancer 1986 (57):197-208

5   Andersson I: Radiographic screening for breast carcinoma. II. Prognostic considerations on the basis of a short-term follow-up. Acta Radiol [Diagn] 1981 (22):227-233

6   Tabár L, Fagerberg CJG, Gad A et al: Reduction in mortality from breast cancer after mass screening with mammography. Lancet 1985 (1):829-832

7   Verbeeck ALM, Hendriks JHCL, Holland R et al: Reduction of breast cancer mortality through mass screening with modern mammography: first results of Nijmegen Project 1975-1981. Lancet 1984 (1):1222-1224

8   Baker LH: Breast cancer detection demonstration project: five year summary report. CA-A Cancer J Clin 1982 (32):194-225

9   Recht A, Danoff BS, Solin LJ et al: Intraductal carcinoma of the breast: results of treatment with excisional biopsy and irradiation. J Clin Oncol 1985 (3):1339-1343

10 Zanfrani B, Fourquet A, Vilcoq JR, Legal M, Calle R: Conservative management of intraductal breast carcinoma with tumorectomy and radiation therapy. Cancer 1986 (57):1299-1301

11 Montague ED: Conservation surgery and radiation therapy in the treatment of operable breast cancer. Cancer 1984 (53-3):700-704

12 Muir R: The evolution of carcinoma of the mamma. J. Pathol 1941 (52):155-172

13 Gallager HS, Martin JE. Early phases in the development of breast cancer. Cancer 1969 (24):1170-1178

14 Helvie MA, Hessler C, Frank TS, Ikeda DM: Atypical hyperplasia of the breast: mammographic appearance and histologic correlation. Radiol 1991 (179):759-764

15 Foote FW, Stewart FW: Lobular carcinoma in situ. A rare form of mammary cancer. Am J Pathol 1941 (17):491-496

16 Wellings SR, Jensen HM: On the origin and progression of ductal carcinoma in the breast. J Natl Cancer Inst 1973 (50):1111-1118

17 McDivitt RW, Stewart FW, Berg JW: Tumors of the breast. In: Firminger HI (ed) Atlas of Tumor Pathology, Armed Forces of Pathology. Washington 1968 pp 22-49

18 Dershaw DD, Abramson A, Kinne DW: Ductal carcinoma in situ: mammographic findings and clinical implications. Radiol 1989 (170):411-415

19 Stomper PC, Connolly JL, Meyer JE, Harris JR: Clinically occult ductal carcinoma in situ detected with mammography: analysis of 100 cases with radiographic-pathologic correlation. Radiol 1989 (172):235-241

20 Patchefsky AS, Schwartz GF, Finkelstein SD et al: Heterogeneity of intraductal carcinoma of the breast. Cancer 1989 (63):731-741

21 Lagios MD: Duct carcinoma in situ. Pathology and treatment. Surg Clin North Am 1990 (70):853-871

22 Andersen J, Blichert-Toft M, Dyreborg U: In situ carcinomas of the breast. Types, growth pattern, diagnosis and treatment. Eur J Surg Onc 1987 (13):105-111

23 Page DL, Dupont WD, Rogers LW, Rados MS: Atypical hyperplasia lesions of the female breast: a long-term follow-up study. Cancer 1985 (55):2698-2708

24 Dupont WD, Page DL: Risk factors for breast cancer in women with proliferative breast disease. N Engl J Med 1985 (312):146-151

25 Cancer Committee of the College of American Pathologists: Is "fibrocystic disease" of the breast precancerous? Arch Pathol Lab Med 1986 (110):171-173

26 Rosai J: Borderline epithelial lesions of the breast. Am J Surg Pathol 1991 (15):209-221

27 Schwartz GF, Patchefsky AS, Finklestein SD et al: Nonpalpable in situ ductal carcinoma of the breast. Predictors of multicentricity and microinvasion and implications for treatment. Arch Surg 1989 (124):29-33

28 Rosen PP, Braun DW, Kinne DE: The clinical significance of pre-invasive breast carcinoma. Cancer 1980 (46):919-925

29 Lagios MD, Margolin FR, Westdahl PR, Rose MR: Mammographically detected duct carcinoma in situ: frequency of local recurrence following tylectomy and prognostic effect of nuclear grade on local recurrence. Cancer 1989 (63):618-624

30 Ringberg A, Palmer B, Linell F: The contralateral breast at reconstructive surgery after breast cancer operation - a histopathological study. Breast Cancer Res Treatment 1982 (2) 151-161

31 Rosen PP, Senie R, Schottenfeld D, Ashikari R: Noninvasive breast carcinoma. Frequency of unsuspected invasion and implications for treatment. Ann Surg 1979 (189):377-382

32 Carter D, Smith RRL: Carcinoma in situ of the breast. Cancer 1977 (40):1189-1193

33 Fentiman IS, Fagg N, Millis RR, Hayward JL: In situ ductal carcinoma of the breast: implications of disease pattern and treatment. Eur J Surg Oncol 1986 (12):261-266

34 Tinnemans JGM, Wobbes T, van der Sluis RF, Lubbers EJC, de Boer HHM: Multicentricity in nonpalpable breast carcinoma and its implications for treatment. Am J Surg 1986 (151):334-338

35 Ciatto S, Grazzini G, Iossa A et al: In situ ductal carcinoma of the breast - analysis of clinical presentation and outcome in 156 consecutive cases. Eur J Surg Oncology 1990 (16):220-224

36 Nielsen M, Thomsen JL, Primdahl S et al: Breast cancer and atypia among young and middle-aged women: a study of 110 medicolegal autopsies. Br J Cancer 1987 (56):814-819

37 Holland R, Hendriks JHCL, Verbeek ALM, Mravunac M, Schuurmans Stekhoven JH: Clinical practice. Extent, distribution, and mammographic/histological correlations of breast ductal carcinoma in situ. Lancet 1990 (335):519-522

38 Lagios MD, Westdahl PR, Margolin FR, Roses MR: Duct carcinoma in situ. Relationship of extent of noninvasive disease to the frequency of occult invasion, multicentricity, lymph node metastases, and shot-term treatment failures. Cancer 1982 (50):1309-1314

39 Ringberg A, Andersson I, Aspegren K, Linell F: Breast carcinoma in situ in 167 women - incidence, mode of presentation, therapy and follow-up. Eur J Surg Oncol 1991 (17):466-476

40 Nielsen M, Jensen J, Andersen J: Precancerous and cancerous breast lesions during lifetime and at autopsy: a study of 83 women. Cancer 1984 (54):612-615

41 Blichert-Toft M, Andersen J, Dyreborg U: Carcinoma in situ mamme. Ugeskr Laeger 1990 (152/25):1803-1806

42 Betsill WL, Rosen PP, Lieberman PH, Robbins FG: Intraductal carcinoma. Long term follow-up after treatment by biopsy alone. JAMA 1978 (239):1863-1867

43 Page DL, Dupont WD, Rogers L, Landenberger M: Intraductal carcinoma of the breast: follow-up after biopsy only. Cancer 1982 (49):751-758

44 Silverstein MJ, Waisman JR, Gamagami P et al: Intraductal carcinoma of the breast (208 cases). Clinical factors influencing treatment choice. Cancer 1990 (66):102-108

45 Zafrani B, Fourquet A, Vilcoq JR, Legal M, Calle R: Conservative management of intraductal breast carcinoma with tumorectory and radiation therapy. Cancer 1986 (57):1299-1301

46 Bornstein BA, Recht A, Connolloy JL et al: Results of treating ductal carcinoma in situ of the breast with conservative surgery and radiation therapy. Cancer 1991 (67):7-13

47 Aasmundstad TA, Haugen OA: DNA ploidy in intraductal breast carcinomas. Eur J Cancer 1990 (26-9):956-959

48 van de Vijver MJ, Peterse JL, Mooi WJ et al: NEU-protein overexpression in breast cancer. Association with comedo-type ductal carcinoma in situ and limited prognostic value in stage II breast cancer. N Engl J Med 1988 (319):1239-1245

49 Meyer JS: Cell kinetics of histologic variants of in situ breast carcinoma. Breast Cancer Res and Treat 1986 (7):171-180

50 Ikeda DM, Andersson I: Ductal carcinoma in situ: atypical mammographic appearances. Radiol 1989 (172):661-666

51 Sigfusson BF, Andersson I, Aspegren K, Janzon L, Linell F, Ljungberg O: Clustered breast calcifications. Acta Radiol (Diagn) 1983 (24):273-281

52 Lanyi M: Diagnosis and Differential Diagnosis of Breast Calcifications. Springer-Verlag, New York 1986 pp 91-107

53 Ahmed A: Calcification in human breast carcinomas: ultrastructural observations. J Pathol 1975 (117):247-251

54 Frappart L, Boudeulle M, Boumendil J et al: Structure and composition of microcalcifications in benign and malignant lesions of the breast: study by light microscopy, transmission and scanning electron microscopy, microprobe analysis, and x-ray diffraction. Hum Pathol 1984 (15):880-889

55 Fandos-Morera A, Prats-Esteve M, Tura-Soteras JM, Traveria-Cros A: Breast tumors: composition of microcalcifications. Radiol 1988 (169):325-327

56 Tornos C, Silva E, El-Naggar A, Pritzker KPH: Calcium oxalate crystals in breast biopsies. The missing calcifications. Am J Surg Pathol 1990 (14-10):961-968

57 Lofgren M, Andersson I, Bondeson L, Linkholm K: X-ray guided fine-needle aspiration for the cytologic diagnosis of nonpalpable breast lesions. Cancer 1988 (61):1032-1037

58 Helvie MA, Baker DE, Adler DD et al: Radiographically guided fine-needle aspiration of non-palpable breast lesions. Radiol 1990 (174):657-661

59 Masood S, Frykberg ER, McLellan GL et al: Prospective evaluation of radiologically directed fine-needle aspiration biopsy of nonpalpable breast lesions. Cancer 1990 (66):1480-1487

60 Sickles EA: Further experience with microfocal spot magnification mammography in the assessment of clustered breast microcalcifications. Radiol 1980 (137):9-14

61 Sickles EA: Mammographic detectability of breast microcalcifications. AJR 1982 (139):913-918

62 Homer MJ: Imaging features and management of characteristically and probably benign breast lesions. Radiol Clin North Am 1987 (25):939-951

63 Sickles EA: Breast calcifications: mammographic evaluation. Radiol 1986 (160):289-293

64 Brenner RS, Sickles EA: Acceptability of periodic follow-up as an alternative to biopsy for mammographically detected lesions interpreted as probably benign. Radiol 1989 (171):645-646

65 Moskowitz M: Impact of a priori medical decisions on screening for breast cancer. Radiol 1989 (171):605-608

66 Hall FM, Storella JM, Silverstone DZ, Wyshak G: Nonpalpable breast lesions: recommendations for biopsy based on suspicion of carcinoma at mammography. Radiol 1988 (167):353-358

Criteria for Recall and Diagnostic Assessment

Stefano Ciattto and Marco Rosselli Del Turco

Centro per lo Studio e la Prevenzione Oncologica, Viale A. Volta 171, 50131 Florence, Italy

Criteria for Recall

Mammographic screening is not aimed at cancer diagnosis, but at the selection of a small subgroup of subjects showing suspicious mammographic abnormalities that require further assessment.

Any recall for a mammographic abnormality, whether subsequently assessed as negative or as benign, must be regarded as inappropriate, since it demonstrates the negative effects of screening and is recorded as a "cost" in the cost/benefit analysis. Unnecessary recall is costly, causes psychological discomfort to the woman and, due to the limited speci-ficity of assessment methods, may produce unnecessary biopsies resulting in further costs, anxiety and diagnostic problems on repeated screening.

Ideally, there should be no unnecessary recall and the positive predictive value for cancer of a recall for further assessment should be 100%. Unfortunately, the specificity of mammography is not very high, in particular for preclinical cancer, which is the main target of screening. As shown in Table 1, the positive predictive value of mammography for preclinical cancer varies according to the radiological appearance of non-palpable lesions but, with the exception of star-like opacities, it is usually less than 50%. In

Table 1. Positive predictive value of different radiological patterns of preclinical lesions at mammography

POSITIVE PREDICTIVE VALUE

| Author [ref] | Opacity | | | | Microcalcifications | | | Distortion |
	Total	Regular	Undefined	Irregular	Total	Low suspect	High suspect	
Bigelow [1]	0.10				0.24			
Ciatto [2]	0.36	0.00	0.35	0.75	0.24	0.02	0.56	0.11
Gisvold [3]	0.25				0.30			
Hall [4]	0.29	0.02		0.93	0.30	0.06	0.34	
Hermann [5]	0.27				0.41			
Lofgren [6]	0.60			0.96	0.31			0.40
Meyer [7]	0.24	0.06	0.15	1.0	0.22			0.29
Schwartz [8]	0.23				0.31			
Silverstein [9]	0.33	0.08	<0.51>		0.25	0.09	0.38	0.10
Tinnemans [10]	0.33	<0.13>		0.67	0.32			

Table 2. Prevalence rates at first screening round in some screening programmes [12]

Study	Age group	No. of cases	Prevalence per 1000 women	Prevalence rate/Annual incidence rate
HIP	40-64	55	2.93	1.30
Sweden	40-49	40	2.15	1.95
	50-59	101	4.63	3.09
	60-69	190	9.08	4.59
Utrecht	50-59	63	6.20	2.95
	60-64	43	9.51	3.80
Florence	40-44	7	0.78	0.76
	45-49	9	2.44	2.51
	50-59	27	4.55	3.14
	60-69	39	8.77	4.82

view of the limited specificity of mammography and their natural concern not to overlook a cancer, radiologists tend to call for investigation even in those cases where radiological abnormality is poorly predictive and a certain number of unnecessary recalls are to be expected.

The classic radiological features giving rise to suspicion on mammography are well known [11], but some cancers have borderline features and a few appear benign. It is difficult, therefore, to establish standard criteria for recall, since the final decision in questionable cases depends on the individual judgement of the radiologist. Periodic comparison with standard reference parameters would be a more reliable method for checking the accuracy of the recall criteria which have been adopted.

Cancer Detection Rate

Although every effort should be made to reduce unnecessary recall rates, it should not cause a reduction in cancer detection rates. The cancer detection rate is the first parameter to be assessed when checking recall criteria. If the detection rate is significantly lower than expected, it means that too strict criteria

for recall have been adopted and that some cancers with atypical borderline features have been reported as negative.

Expected detection rates vary according to the age-specific incidence and the prevalence/estimated incidence ratio is a good indicator of early detection. As shown in Table 2, prevalence (detection rate at first screening) and prevalence/incidence ratios are similar in different programmes: when women over 50 are screened the first time round, a standard detection rate of >5 per thousand and a prevalence/incidence ratio of >3 seem to constitute a reasonable reference standard.

The cancer detection rate will, of course, drop when screening is repeated and the estimated rate varies according to the re-screening interval. As shown in Table 3, a detection rate of about 3% may be taken as a reference standard with a 2-year re-screening interval.

Double reading seems to be a good tool for increasing the sensitivity of screening, particularly when carried out by newly trained radiologists. Such a hypothesis is confirmed by preliminary findings reported by a few screening programmes (Edinburgh, Strasbourg and Florence); further evaluation is needed, however, and the opposite effect of an increased recall rate has to be assessed.

Table 3. Cancer detection rates (per 1000 examined) at repeated screening in women aged 50 or more

Programme	[ref]	First screening (per thousand)	Repeated screening (per thousand)
Florence (1975-86)	[12]	3.3	6.4
Nijmegen (1975-86)	[13]	5.6	4.9
Utrecht (1974-80)	[14]	7.2	1.9
Edinburgh (1979-87)*	[15]	6.1	3.2

* age 45-64

Recall Rates

Provided that the above-mentioned reference standard is achieved, recall rates should be the lowest possible. As shown in Table 4, recall rates are constantly below 5% on first screening. When screening is repeated, previous mammographies are available for review and many suspicious findings are thus ruled out. Repeated screening has shown that recall rates are constantly lower, usually below 2%: therefore, a maximum recall rate of 5% at the first screening and 2% at a further screening seem to be a reasonable reference standard.

When recall rates are higher than the reference standards, it means that the criteria adopted for recall are too extensive and that too many subjects have been recalled due to false mammographic reports. In such an event, the recalled cases should be reviewed and the positive predictive value for cancer should be determined for each category of mammographic abnormality. This will permit poorly predictive patterns to be identified and new recall criteria to be adopted.

As mentioned above, double reading may increase the recall rate, but its extent has not been definitely assessed. Another factor

Table 4. Recall rates at first or repeated screening of women aged 50 or more

Programme	[ref]	First screening (percent)	Repeated screening (percent)
Florence (1987-89)	[16]	2.3	1.1
Nijmegen (1975-86)	[13]	1.5	0.9
Utrecht (1974-80)	[14]	3.3	1.6

which may increase the recall rate is the use of the single oblique view.

It is well known that many asymmetric opacities or parenchymal distortions may show false images due to superimposition, whereas if the craniocaudal view is available, lesions can be recognised easily.

Assessment Modalities

Recall for assessment is the last step of the screening procedure marking the beginning of the diagnostic phase. Women are recalled to the assessment unit, where possible, by way of a computerised system. Non-compliers should be informed of the possible consequences of not complying and every effort should be made to convince them to accept the assessment procedure.

The assessment unit should be in a centralised location and should be supervised under the screening programme. There should be a multidisciplinary team, the members of which are both expert and experienced: these teams should include clinicians, radiologists, cytologists and pathologists who should all have had specific training in breast cancer diagnosis.

Mammography

Additional mammographic views, or direct magnification, are often performed for a better evaluation of abnormalities seen on the screening films. Magnification requires a microfocus (0.1 mm) mammographic unit and is particularly useful for the detailed analysis of microcalcifications.

Physical Examination

This is mandatory in the presence of subjective symptoms (mass, discharge), or of a mammographic abnormality which has not been ruled out by subsequent views. It must be carried out by a trained clinician, but not necessarily a surgeon.

Sonography

High frequency (7.5-10 MHz) and small parts focussed probes must be employed. Sonography is highly specific in differentiating solid from cystic lesions, especially when dealing with preclinical lesions and it may improve the differential diagnosis of palpable masses in very dense breasts.

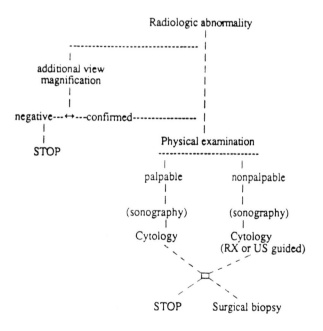

Fig. 1. Flow chart of the assessment procedure

Cytology

All lesions for which even a minimal suspicion of cancer arises on mammography, physical examination or sonography, either palpable or non-palpable, should undergo fine-needle aspiration cytology. Aspiration should be performed by trained operators using the correct techniques with low inadequacy rates [17]. Sonographic or radiological (stereotaxic) guidance is required for non-palpable lesions and these procedures must be performed by experienced radiologists.

All these facilities must be available at the assessment unit and should be carried out during a single session in order to keep the anguish and discomfort of the patient and loss of time to a minimum. A flow chart of the assessment policy is shown in Figure 1.

Tables 5 and 6 show the preliminary assessment results of cases selected by the mammographic screening programme that was recently launched in the city of Florence, Italy. As shown in Table 5, the predictive value of call for biopsy following diagnostic assessment is 90%: 2 out of 3 false-positive cases were reported on the basis of irregular microcalcifications and 1 case of cancer was diagnosed by positive cytology in a round opacity with a regular outline. The contribution of different assessment tests to the avoidance of surgical biopsy in the remaining 179 cases is analysed in Table 6: in 50% of the cases the mammographic indication had disappeared or had been judged as benign following assessment mammography and no further investigation was considered necessary. Sonography also made a significant contribution, whereas negative cytology was a determining factor in 10% of the cases.

The aim of assessment is to separate those lesions which are most probably benign and do not require a biopsy from those in which the risk of malignancy is sufficiently high as to justify surgery. Thus, the accuracy of the assessment procedure may be monitored through the biopsy rate, provided that the cancer detection rate is consistent with the previously indicated standard reference and the benign/malignant ratio (B/M). As shown in Table 7, the biopsy rate and the B/M have changed significantly over a period of time. This change can probably be attributed to the

Table 5. Florence city project. Preliminary results on diagnostic assessment (20/9/90 - 30/5/91). Mammographic pattern by diagnostic conclusion after assessment

| | Diagnostic conclusion | | | | | |
| | *Control* | | *Biopsy* | | | |
Mammographic pattern	2 years	1 year	Benign (histology)	Carcinoma (histology)	Total	Row %
No RX signs (symptoms)	5	-	-	-	5	2.4
Regular opacity	27	4	0	1	32	15.3
Irregular opacity	60	15	1	16	92	44.0
Distortion	23	2	0	1	26	12.4
Microcalcification	14	18	2	9	43	20.6
Asymmetry	11	-	-	-	11	5.3
Total	140	39	3	27	209	100
Col. %	67.0	18.7	1.4	12.9		

increasing experience of the operators and the greater accuracy of the assessment procedure. The biopsy rate will be higher and the predictive value of a biopsy will be lower at first when compared with repeated screening. At the first screening, the biopsy rate should be around 1% and the B/M should be at least 1:1 (predictive value 50%). On repeated

Table 6. Florence city project. Preliminary results on diagnostic assessment (20/9/90 - 30/5/91). Diagnostic tests which avoided biopsy by mammographic pattern

Mammographic pattern	X-ray detailed examination	Palpation	Echography	Cytology	Total row %
No radiological sign (symptoms)	-	5	-	-	2.8
Regular opacity	4	6	15	6	17.3
Irregular opacity	42	10	17	6	41.9
Distortion	21	2	2	-	-
Microcalcifications	19	3	5	5	17.9
Asymmetric density	3	3	4	1	6.1
Total	73	29	43	18	
Col. %	49.7	16.2	24.0	10.1	

Table 7. Biopsy rate (per 100 screening examinations) and biopsy positive predictive value (PVV) or B/M ratio

Programme [ref]	Biopsy rate	PPV	B/M ratio
Florence [16]			
(1979-81)	0.9%	0.33	2:1
(1982-84)	0.9%	0.32	2:1
(1985-86)	0.6%	0.48	1:1
(1987-89)	0.3%	0.92	1:11
Nijmegen [3]			
1st round	0.9%	0.51	1:1
2nd round	0.4%	0.69	1:2.3
3rd round	0.4%	0.62	1:1.7
4th round	0.3%	0.71	1:2.5
5th round	0.4%	0.87	1:7
6th round	0.3%	0.97	1:32

Table 8. Benign to malignant biopsy ratio (B/M). Consecutive series of non-palpable lesions where stereotaxic (or US guided) cytology was not routinely employed

Author	Cases	B/M
Abel et al. 1988	152	4.4:1
Arnesson et al. 1986	314	1.5:1
Bigelow et al. 1985	150	5.2:1
Ciatto et al. 1987	512	2.4:1
Dershaw 1986	219	2.5:1
Gisvold & Martin 1984	343	2.7:1
Graham & Bauer 1988	678	7.7:1
Hall et al. 1988	400	2.4:1
Hermann et al. 1987	220	1.9:1
Marrujo et al. 1986	237	2.7:1
Meyer et al. 1984	500	3.3:1
Ostrow et al. 1987	121	7.1:1
Poole et al. 1986	148	6.0:1
Schwartz et al. 1988	1132	2.4:1
Silverstein et al. 1987	653	3.4:1
Skinner et al. 1988	179	3.4:1
Stock et al. 1989	280	5.2:1
Tinnemans et al. 1987	359	2.0:1
Wilhelm et al. 1986	452	3.8:1
Yankaskas et al. 1988	199	5.2:1
Total	7248	3.0:1

Modified from Ciatto [22]

screening reference standards of 0.5% for the biopsy rate and 1:2 for B/M seem reasonable. Most calls for surgical biopsy at assessment are due to suspected non-palpable lesions. In the 1970s, when stereotaxic or US-guided cytology was not routinely available, the final decision on biopsy was based on the mammographic appearance and, due to the limited specificity of mammography (see Table 1), the B/M for non-palpable lesions was rather high; 3:1 on average (see Table 8). When cytology was currently available, it helped the final decision concerning biopsy. As false negatives are expected, the call for a surgical biopsy, due to strong suspicion aroused by mammography, will not be contraindicated by a negative cytological report, but when suspicion is moderate, a plain negative cytological report will reassure the radiologist, who will decide to follow-up the case instead of advising a biopsy. This policy does not seem to reduce cancer detection rates [18] and has a highly favourable impact on the B/M, which, in all the cases where stereotaxic cytology was employed, dropped below 1:1 (see Table 9). Thus, the routine use of cytology is recommended for non-palpable lesions. A certain number of cases can be managed by sonographically-guided aspiration, which is simpler, cheaper and quicker than stereotaxic procedures, but about half the cases worth a cytological assessment, especially isolated calcifications (see Table 10), are not visible to sonography and thus a stereotaxic facility should be available at the assessment unit.

Table 9. Benign to malignant biopsy ratio (B/M). Consecutive series of non-palpable lesions where stereotaxic (or US guided) cytology was routinely employed

Author [ref]	Cases	B/M
Azavedo [19]	567	1:3.1
Ciatto [18]	115	1:1.8
Lofgren [20]	103	1:1.6

Table 10. Distribution of 117 consecutive non-palpable lesions by radiological appearance and aspiration modality (sonography-guided or stereotaxic). Florence, 1990-91

Radiological appearance	Aspiration modality	
	US-guided	Stereotaxic
Opacity with sharp or poorly defined borders	61	8
Star-like opacity	6	6
Distortion	1	4
Isolated calcifications	13	78
Total	81	96

Surgical biopsy is the final assessment modality in suspected cases. There is much discussion as to whether general anaesthesia or local anaesthesia (when possible) should be adopted and whether frozen biopsy with immediate treatment or a two-step procedure (excisional biopsy and standard histopathological evaluation on inclusion) should be employed [21], but this controversy seems unresolved to date.

As far as non-palpable lesions are concerned, preoperative localisation by the injection of a suspension of medical carbon or by positioning a hook-wire, is mandatory. The former method is more practical as it can be routinely performed at the time of stereotaxic cytology (the trace persists for months), whereas the hook-wire is positioned 1 or 2 days before surgery and must be removed surgically. Perioperative mammography of the surgical specimen is also necessary in order to assess the adequate removal of the lesion. It is recommended that surgical biopsies be performed by surgeons having specific experience in the management of non-palpable lesions.

REFERENCES

1   Bigelow R, Smith R, Goodman PA and Wilson GS: Needle localization of nonpalpable breast masses. Arch Surg 1985 (120):565-569

2   Ciatto S, Cataliotti L and Distante V: Nonpalpable lesions detected with mammography: review of 512 consecutive cases. Radiol 1987 (165):99-102

3   Gisvold JJ and Martin JK: Prebiopsy localization of nonpalpable breast lesions. AJR 1984 (143):477-481

4   Hall FM, Storella JM, Silverston DZ and Wyshak G: Nonpalpable breast lesions: recommendations for biopsy based on suspicion of carcinoma at mammography. Radiol 1988 (167):353-358

5   Hermann G, Janus C, Schwartz IS, Krivisky B, Bier S and Rabinowitz JG: Nonpalpable breast lesions: accuracy of prebiopsy mammographic diagnosis. Radiol 1987 (165):323-326

6   Lofgren M, Andersson I, Bondeson L and Lindholm K: X-ray guided fine needle aspiration for the cytologic diagnosis of nonpalpable breast lesions. Cancer 1988 (61):1032-1037

7   Meyer JE, Kopans DB, Stomper PC and Lindfors KK: Occult breast abnormalities: percutaneous preoperative needle localization. Radiol 1984 (150):335-337

8   Schwartz GF, Feig SA and Patchefsky AS: Significance and staging of nonpalpable carcinomas of the breast. Surg Gynecol Obstet 1988 (166):6-10

9   Silverstein MJ, Gamagami P, Rosser RJ, Gierson ED, Colburn WJ, Handel N, Fingerhut AG, Lewinsky BS, Hoffman RS and Waisman JR: Hooked-wire directed breast biopsy and overpenetrated mammography. Cancer 1987 (59):715-722

10 Tinnemans JGM, Wobbes T, Holland R, Hendriks JHCL, van der Sluis RF, Lubbers EJC and de Boer HHM: Mammmographic and histopathologic correlation of nonpalpable lesions of the breast and the reliability of frozen section diagnosis. Surg Gynecol Obstet 1987 (165):523-529

11 Tabar L: Atlas of Mammography. Springer Verlag, Berlin 1983

12 Paci E, Ciatto S, Buiatti E, Cecchini S, Palli D and Rosselli Del Turco M: Early indicators of efficacy of breast cancer screening programmes. Results of the Florence district programme. Int J Cancer 1990 (46):198-202

13 Peeters PHM, Verbeek ALM, Hendriks JHCL and van Bon MJH: Screening for breast cancer in Nijmegen. Report of 6 screening rounds, 1975-1986. Int J Cancer 1989 (437):226-230

14 De Waard F, Collette HJA, Rombach JJ, Baanders-van Halewijn EA and Honig C: The DOM project for the early detection of breast cancer, Utrecht, The Netherlands. J Chron Dis 1984 (37):1-44

15 Roberts RR, Alexander FE, Anderson TJ, Chetty U, Donnan PT, Forrest P, Hepburn W, Huggins A, Kirkpatrick AE, Lamb J, Muir BB and Prescott RJ: Edinburgh trial of screening for breast cancer: mortality at seven years. Lancet 1990 (i):241-246

16 Ciatto S and Rosselli Del Turco M: Tassi di richiamo per approfondimento e per invio a biopsia chirurgica a seguito di screening mammografico. Radiol Med 1991 (82):56-59

17 Ciatto S, Catania S, Bravetti P, Bonardi R, Cariaggi P and Pacifico E: Fine-needle cytology of the breast: a controlled study of aspiration versus nonaspiration. Diag Cytopath 1991 (7):125-127

18 Ciatto S, Rosselli Del Turco M and Bravetti P: Nonpalpable breast lesions: stereotaxic fine-needle aspiration cytology. Radiol 1989 (173):57-59

19 Azavedo E, Svane G and Auer G: Stereotactic fine-needle biopsy in 2594 mammographically detected non-palpable lesions. Lancet 1989 (i):1033-1035

20 Lofgren M, Andersson I and Lindholm K: Stereotactic fine-needle aspiration for cytologic diagnosis of nonpalpable breast lesions. AJR 1989 (154):1191-1195

21 Forrest APM: The surgeon's role in breast screening. World J Surg 1989 (13):19-24

22 Ciatto S: Diagnosi differenziale del cancro non palpabile della mammella. In: Cataliotti L, Ciatto S, Luini A (eds) Le Neoplasie Precliniche della Mammella. Sorbona, Milano 1990 pp 13-30

Pathology in Breast Cancer Screening: A 15-Year Experience from a Swedish Programme

Adel Gad

Department of Clinical Pathology and Cytology, Falun Hospital, 79182 Falun, Sweden

The Swedish "Two-County" breast cancer screening programme has often been described in the literature, most recently in January 1992 [1]. Screening was set up in Kopparberg County in October 1977 and in Ostergötland in May 1978. After completing 4 rounds of screening in women aged 40 to 49 years, 3 rounds in those between the ages of 50 and 69 and 2 in the age group from 70 to 74, screening in the control group was initiated in Kopparberg in 1984. Since 1987, all women between the ages of 40 to 69 are being invited to 2-view mammography at 20-month intervals, the ultimate aim being to reduce this interval to 18 months in the 40-49 age group.

Two decades of the widespread use of mammography has impacted profoundly on the diagnosis, management, and outcome of breast cancer. Many of the detected lesions are impalpable, clinically occult and to be seen in asymptomatic women. In the light of the diversity of options open for managing patients with premalignant and malignant lesions, it is becoming ever more imperative to counsel patients individually on the choice of the most satisfactory treatment. Consequently, quantitative and qualitative changes have been made in breast pathology procedures and established policies and techniques have undergone major revision.

The Multidisciplinary Team Approach

In the past, the pathologist was called upon to answer the simple question of whether the mass was benign or malignant and often to confirm a clinical diagnosis. His skill was rarely challenged further and the therapeutic alternatives were limited.

Within a screening programme today, he is a partner in a multidisciplinary team and is required to furnish information concerning the exact nature of the disease.

This entails cytological and histological data when assessing clinically occult lesions revealed in mammography, such as microcalcifications, architectural distortion and asymmetric densities. In the increasing number of borderline cases, the pathologist should be able to make accurate diagnoses, including the prognostic criteria on which proper management is based. All the information collected should be used to create a database by which the outcome of the screening programme can be monitored. The pathologist should be familiar with the techniques required for handling surgical specimens and diagnosing subtle lesions. Most pathologists are familiar with and competent in dealing with problems concerning symptomatic breast disease. However, only few of them will be prepared, without further education and training, to take the responsibilities created by screening asymptomatic women. The pathologist should also be familiar with the radiological appearances of breast lesions and be acquainted with the recent developments in the management of breast cancer. Other members of the team should also acquire knowledge of the anatomic and cytopathological basis of breast disease.

Members of the multidisciplinary team are to be aware of the possibilities offered by and the limitations encountered in the usage of screening test, mammography, diagnostic method, histopathology, as well as aspiration cytology which is mainly employed in the assessment of recalled patients. A proper and rational use of these procedures will cause mammographic screening to be both optimal and cost effective. Newly detected cases will undergo at least 2 stages of discussion and decision making - the mammographer will have sole responsibility for selection of women to undergo further mammographic, clinical and/or cytological assessment. After careful consideration by the team [2,3], the surgeon will select cases for primary or definitive surgery and the final diagnosis will be made by the pathologist. The management of these cases will then be the responsibility of the entire team who, at regular meetings, will base their decisions on carefully defined protocols [3].

To be effective, a screening programme should achieve a balance between the number of occult cancers detected and the number of women recalled for assessment on the one hand, and the number of surgical operations carried out for malignant lesions and those for benign lesions on the other. A malignant lesion missed will reappear at the next screening, or between screens, at a more advanced stage, with the potential risk of doing nothing to reduce mortality from breast cancer, whereas recalling women for reassessment unnecessarily and submitting them to surgery for benign lesions will undermine both the cost-effectiveness and confidence in screening. Management and follow-up of women with cancer or precancerous lesions should be tailored, on an individual basis, according to the nature and extent of the disease present. In the long run, the value of screening will be judged on whether breast cancer mortality does actually show a reduction [4].

Pathology with its 2 main arms, cytopathology and histopathology, is basic to screening and the achievement of its objectives. The changing role of the pathologist within these programmes has been the subject of many guidelines representing the prevailing views and attitudes in diverse institutions [5] and national [6-8] and European organisations [9]. Three review articles on this subject were published recently [10-12]. Such a diversity of approach to the demands of the new situation reflects the complexity of this issue and the way different programmes are organised and conducted. Understandably, experience cannot be replicated exactly. However, on the basis of 15 years' experience in specialist centres, general agreement has been reached concerning technical methods and diagnosis which give consistently good results. Based on pathological procedures adopted in the ongoing screening programme in the Swedish county of Kopparberg, this chapter will present recommendations for training and programme strategies which could be used as guidelines despite existing differences in national cyto-histopathological procedures and organisation.

The Work Load

From the point of view of quality, screening for breast cancer changes the spectrum of lesions and the panorama of histological findings. The so-called grey zone or borderland in diagnostic breast pathology, the area between clear-cut malignant and benign, in which subtle, borderline and cancer-mimicking lesions find their place, is widened. This issue will not be addressed in this chapter.

From the point of view of quantity, screening has increased the work load due, first of all, to a sharp rise in the number of breast preparations and to the adoption of more sophisticated, time-consuming techniques.

During the first round of screening, the "prevalence screen", between 1977 and 1980, the number of surgical specimens increased by almost 44% as compared with 1976 (Fig. 1), and it decreased gradually to just above pre-screening levels during the second round between 1983-1985. A steady figure almost similar to that of pre-screening levels was reached when screening of the whole female population between 40 and 69 years was repeated.

The number of cytological examinations varied widely in the different rounds of screening, increasing in relation to 1967 by 25% and 73% in 1982 and 1985, respectively. The sharp rise in 1985 was partly due to both study and control groups being screened simultaneously and partly to a deviation from the original policy on the use of cytology, described later on in this chapter.

A study was carried out by the Pathology Department of the Royal Liverpool University Hospital [13] on the influence on the work load of the differences in handling screening and non-screening excision biopsy specimens. Methods recommended for processing excision biopsy specimens from patients in the screening programme led to a significantly higher number of blocks being initially taken as compared with those taken from patients who had not been screened (8.03 vs 4.95; p=0.000001). The same increase was noted when only the malignant cases were compared (7.74 vs 6.02; p=0.00014).

A comparison of the demand for surgical inpatient care between 1974 and 1983 in the counties of Kopparberg and Uppsala was carried out [14]. There was no mass screening programme in Uppsala county. An increase of some 150% in surgery and days of hospital care required for breast cancer patients was observed in Kopparberg during the initial round, the numbers falling during the second and third rounds to those of the control group. The sharp increase in the surgical work load was observed mainly in the 50-69 age group, whereas in the 40-49 age group little extra demand was made on resources.

Pathological and surgical work loads are, thus, dependent on the length of the screening period and the age range of the population invited.

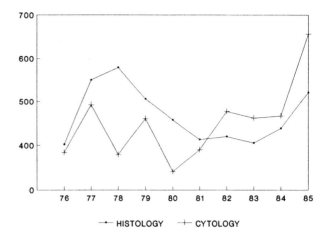

Fig. 1. The number of histological and cytological examinations perfomed at the Department of Pathology, Falun Hospital, 1976-1985

who will be diagnosed accurately with the minimum number of open biopsies.

The first round of screening in our county produced the following figures: 94.8% in the 40-69 age group (31,094) proved normal after single-view mammography [15]. Assessment with additional mammographic views, spot compression views, microfocus magnification, pneumocystography and/or galactography were performed, as required, in 5.2% (1,606 women). The suspected abnormality was not confirmed in 3.4% (1,053), 1.8% (553) were given physical and/or cytological examination of whom 0.9% (285) were referred for open biopsy. Histologically proven carcinoma was observed in 0.5% (156) cases.

Preoperative Assessment and Diagnostic Work-Up

About 40% of all cancers [14] and many of the atypical and cancer-mimicking benign abnormalities are picked up by mammography in the occult, clinically impalpable state during a screening programme. Preoperative assessment and diagnostic work-up require the application of a number of sophisticated procedures (complete mammography with pneumocystography and galactography, clinical and cytological examinations) in order to obtain the maximum number of women

Needle Biopsy Techniques

Needle biopsy techniques include fine-needle aspiration cytology (FNAC) and core biopsy (CB) which can both be performed in the out-patient clinic.

Fine-Needle Aspiration Cytology

Originating in the 1930s at the Memorial Sloan-Kettering Cancer Center, New York, it was adopted and developed in the 1960s at the Radiumhemmet, Karolinska Hospital, in

Stockholm, Sweden [16,17]. Since it had been used extensively throughout Sweden, when mammographic screening was initiated on a national basis, it was found that, contrary to the situation in the United States and the United Kingdom, there was no shortage of qualified cytologists in the country, where most cytologists are also histopathologists. In view of the close and synergistic relationship between histo- and cytopathology, it is preferable that the cytologist also practises histopathology.

FNAC is seen to be a simple, safe, cost effective and reliable tool in the assessment of palpable lesions of the breast which, when used in combination with mammographic and clinical examination - the so-called triple approach - can achieve a diagnostic accuracy of over 99% [18]. In our screening programme, when all 3 modalities indicated a cancer diagnosis in palpable abnormalities, the definitive therapeutic surgery was carried out without any further histological proof of malignancy. If full preoperative diagnostic agreement was not achieved, definitive therapy was preceded either by frozen section or open biopsy.

Used mainly to confirm a diagnosis of cancer in palpable lesions, it is used also to confirm diagnosis in benign lesions, in which case, however, FNAC has the added property of reducing the number of open biopsies. Aspiration of non-palpable abnormalities will, therefore, require extremely accurate, image-guided needle placement: X-ray [19], including stereotaxis, coordinated grid and perforated plate, ultrasound devices [20] or computed tomography [21] being the methods adopted to ensure precision. Indications for mammographically-guided FNAC of non-palpable lesions include clustered microcalcifications, ill-defined or spiculated densities, solitary or newly developed well-defined masses and, less frequently, focal architectural distortions [20].

Reports in the literature showed that the discriminatory power of diagnosing benign and malignant breast disease [22] revealed striking dissimilarities in the probability of obtaining a precise FNAC outcome. This was due to 3 main factors: the quality of FNAC being distinctly operator-dependent provides a psychological reason for publication bias, as poor test quality indicates poor human performance; details of size and type of tumours were scanty; in the process of calculating sensitivity and specificity, any inadequate, unsatisfactory or sparse specimens were considered either negative, or were discarded.

This practice of discarding inadequate specimens is regarded as highly deplorable as it will lead to results which do not reflect the true performance of the technique in everyday routine, and overestimate its usefulness [20,22]. Rates of inadequacy vary from 1.3% [23] to 36.3% [24], as shown in Table 1, whereas the impact of excluding inadequate specimens on sensitivity and specificity rates, as calculated by Fornage [20], is shown in Table 2. Inadequate cytology will more likely be obtained from a benign lesion (21-42%) than from a carcinoma (8-17%) [24,27].

Optimal use of a diagnostic tool requires knowledge not only of how accurate it is but also of its limitations [24]. One of the major limitations to the use of FNAC for impalpable lesions are the unacceptably high figures of false-negative and false-positive results [28]. Where stereotaxic FNAC was originally developed and extensively used [26], the rate of inadequate and false-negative results amounted to 33.6% and that of false positives to 10.1%. Variations in these rates as reported in the literature are partly due to differences in the way results are analysed and expressed. Suspicious reports are sometimes considered as positive and sometimes as negative, and the overall accuracy might be expressed as that of both benign and malignant lesions, or only in the diagnosis of carcinoma [20,22].

False-negative results are significantly higher

Table 1. The rate of sparse and inadequate aspiration cytology material in various screening programmes

Programme	Rate of inadequate material
Linköping [23]	1.3%
Stockholm [25,26]	7.5%, 8.6%
Florence [27]	16.5%
Malmö [24]	36.3%

Table 2. The effect of exclusion of inadequate cytological specimens on sensitivity and specificity in two screening programmes

Paper	No. of lesions	No. of cancers	Inadequate specimens	Sensitivity Orig.*	Rev.**	Specificity Orig.	Rev.
Ciatto et al. [27]	218	74	36 (16.5%)	84%	77%	97%	76%
Löfgren et al. [24]	215	47	78 (36.3%)	92%	77%	95%	NA***

* original ** revised *** not available

for impalpable lesions when compared with FNAC of palpable abnormalities [29] due to the small size and fibrous content of some lesions, or the potential for sampling error, the so-called geographic miss. This can be due to the wide area occupied by the lesion, or to the complex nature of the abnormality comprising both benign and malignant structures. An additional factor for X-ray guided stereotaxic technique is that it is not possible to vary the angle through which the needle penetrates the lesion during sampling [29]. For these reasons, multiple sampling is recommended, occasionally up to 5 [29] or more [23] separate punctures to increase the diagnostic yield.

Another major limitation to the use of FNAC in the assessment of impalpable lesions is that even an unequivocal cancer diagnosis cannot differentiate between invasive and non-invasive carcinoma and should not, purely on its own merits, lead to definitive surgery. This clearly contradicts what has been claimed by some workers in the field that one of the main advantages of cancer cytology in impalpable lesions is that it results in one-stage cancer surgery [23,24,26,29]. Detailed histopathological information should be provided prior to the proper management on an individual basis. This information should include the basic characteristics of the tumour nature, type, size and extent as well as its nuclear grade, degree of differentiation and the margins of excision. The final arbiter in the diagnosis of an impalpable lesion and its eventual management must be a full and thorough histological assessment. This policy agrees with the guidelines for cytopathologists as laid down in Britain and Sweden [29,30]. The British guidelines state that no cytology find-

ings for impalpable lesions should be interpreted in isolation, negative reports should be viewed with caution and, in most cases, confirmed by open biopsy [29]. Under no circumstances should a cytological opinion of malignancy in the absence of mammographic and/or clinical evidence be taken as authority to proceed to therapeutic surgery. The Swedish guidelines go further, stating that even in the case of positive cytology, the suspicious area should be excised with a wide free margin and subjected to histopathological examination before mastectomy and/or axillary clearance [30].

The latter document, in fact, recommends, when required, double cytological reading, in both palpable and impalpable lesions. Due to the limitations already discussed, FNAC was not used in our programme until 1985 on lesions measuring 10 mm or less in diameter or on any group of microcalcifications. These lesions were excised in toto, on pure mammographic evaluation and examined histologically, following preoperative needle localisation. Table 3 illustrates the impact of this strategy on the benign/malignant ratio in Kopparberg as compared to the South Hospital in Stockholm where FNAC was used for all types of lesions [31]. A slightly higher benign to malignant ratio, within acceptable limits, is shown to result in a higher share of detected cancers. In our programme, FNAC was used after 1985 for some impalpable cases without significantly altering this ratio.

Clearly, FNAC will have beneficial effects where the standards of mammographic screening are not high [29,32]. Nevertheless, cytology should not be used in screening programmes to compensate for unsatisfactory

Table 3. Comparison between the course of events during preoperative assessment in two Swedish projects of mammographic screening (%)

Round of screening	Screening project	Abnormal findings		Referred to surgery	Benign/Malignant ratio	
		after SVM	after CM			
First	Kopparberg [15]	5.2	1.8	0.9	0.4	0.5
	Stockholm [31]	5.1	1.5	0.6	0.2	0.4
Second	Kopparberg	3.0	0.9	0.5	0.2	0.4
	Stockholm	3.2	0.8	0.4	0.1	0.3

SVM = single-view mammography; CM = complete mammography

mammographic results, standards should be optimal and mammography should yield as few false-positive results as possible.

The answer to the question who performs aspiration depends largely on how each programme is organised and conducted. Usually aspiration of palpable lesions is performed by clinicians or cytopathologists and by mammographers if it is X-ray or ultrasound guided. The result of cytological examination should be made available without delay, if requested, during the assessment process. However, no pressure should be used to provide a diagnosis if the cytopathologist is uncertain.

Stereotaxic Core Biopsy

In view of the limitations of FNAC, particularly the high rate of inadequate material and failure to differentiate between *in-situ* and infiltrative carcinoma, the search for a supplementary procedure for preoperative evaluation of impalpable abnormalities has led to the successful tissue sampling by stereotaxic large-core (14 gauge) biopsies developed over the last 3 years by Steve Parker and his co-workers in the US [33,34]. A diagnostic accuracy equivalent to surgical excision has been reported. Our experience over the last 12 months confirms that of others, both in America and elsewhere [35,36]. This procedure is indicated for sampling small, solitary, multiple solid or cystic masses and in selected cases of microcalcifications. Stereotaxic core biopsy (SCB) should not replace other methods but complement them.

FNAC, SCB and excisional biopsy should be used in a complementary and uncompetitive manner in the investigation and diagnosis of mammographically-detected abnormalities. SCB is superior in non-palpable mammographically malignant stellate and benign circular lesions, whereas FNAC may be helpful in circular malignant abnormalities.

Preoperative Localisation and Specimen Radiography

Many of the cancers diagnosed by mammography are occult and have to be localised by preoperative radiography and perioperative specimen radiography, preferably with the close cooperation of the mammographer and the surgeon. The precise location and depth of the abnormality are indicated by the mammographer, thus enabling the surgeon to remove the area occupied by the lesion.

Various methods have been used which include skin markers, dye injections, needles, and hooked wires. Injection of an aqueous suspension of medical carbon has been used in association with stereotaxic fine-needle aspiration to mark impalpable lesions [37]. The hook-wire technique, introduced in 1976 [38], has proved to be very satisfactory. We use ordinary spinal needles to insert home-made wires.

The importance of specimen radiography for clinically impalpable abnormalities seen as suspicious on mammography is generally recognised [39,40]. After mammography of the specimen with the wire in place and removal of the lesion in question, the fresh specimen will be sent intact to the pathologist together with the radiogram and the mammographer's report. The specimen should be marked in such a way as to enable the pathologist to make the proper orientation. Macroscopic examination and palpation alone do not allow the pathologist to perform adequate sampling and to choose the correct slices of the operative specimen.

The specimen should be cut into thin slices, about 0.5 cm thick, arranged in sequence on a clean radiographic film, after which they will be numbered. Another radiograph will be taken. The slices representing the lesion seen in the original mammogram should be selected by the mammographer before being processed at the pathology department.

Specimen radiography can also be useful for sampling mastectomy specimens. The breast is placed with the skin surface on the cut-up board and the quadrants are cut into 0.5 cm thick slices. The slices from each quadrant will be placed on a clean radiography film, numbered and sent for radiography.

When reviewing slides from operation specimens taken because of microcalcifications, it is important to make sure that these calcifications are visualised in the sections. Failure to do this should lead to cutting additional sections from the block. In some cases, it is necessary to turn to paraffin block radiography to identify the calcifications. This procedure should be followed thoroughly by the pathologist and continued until both he and the mammographer are completely convinced that the abnormality in question has been fully examined [41]. The choice of apparatus and the location for specimen radiography depends upon the local working conditions. We prefer the specimen radiography to be performed by the mammographer using the screening equipment. In other screening settings, small self-contained units placed in the department of pathology have been used [10,42].

Frozen Section Diagnosis

This is a highly reliable procedure in the diagnosis of carcinoma in both palpable and impalpable breast lesions [43-45]. It is only valuable, however, when it answers the question of whether or not the surgeon must proceed to mastectomy - a situation rarely met within screening as it does not provide the magnitude of information on which modern management is based. In agreement with many others, we concur that frozen section diagnosis is not appropriate in the examination of impalpable abnormalities [5,7,10-12,45-47] because of diagnostic and sampling limitations.

Differentiating between the many types of subtle breast lesions is already difficult, diagnosis by way of permanent paraffin sections is often made even more difficult due to the initial freezing of the tissue which causes distortion or destruction of the specimen and frozen section does not allow either for the pathologist to consult about diagnosis alternatives, or for the patient to be counselled concerning therapy options.

The Two-Stage Procedure

The one-stage procedure has long been standard for both diagnosing and treating breast cancer [48] and frozen section was an essential part of this procedure. In recent years, conservative surgery has become the norm for certain cases of breast cancer and frozen section has rarely been used since. For lesions of 10 mm in diameter or smaller, or cases of mammographically suspicious microcalcifications, diagnostic segmentectomy rather than simple tumour excision has been used.

After thorough histopathological examination, this procedure can prove satisfactory as a therapeutic measure, or a second stage entailing axillary dissection, wider resection or mastectomy may be performed. Segmentectomy is a strictly standardised, well-defined sector-like resection of tissue from the centre to the periphery of the tumour bearing part of the breast [49,50]. The 2-stage procedure was adopted in our county in 1981 and can offer many advantages [51]; a thorough histopathological examination is decisive for its success in achieving the therapeutic goal of local tumour control.

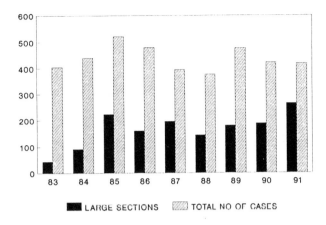

Fig. 2. The number of large sections prepared at the department of pathology, Falun Hospital, in relation to the total number of cases from 1983 to 1991

Examination of Surgical Specimens and Sampling Strategies

One of the most serious problems facing pathologists involved in breast cancer screening is the absence of generally accepted guidelines on what should be a proper histopathological examination of the surgical specimens.

There is general consensus on the extent of information that should be passed on to the other members of the multidisciplinary team, but there is great diversity with regard to the extent to which the resected breast tissue should be sampled and the resection margins examined [10,12]. The extent of sampling varies from examining only the area of the specimen containing the mammographic abnormality to submitting a variable amount of the remaining tissue for microscopic examination.

However, no matter what size the specimen should be, it has been established that histological examination of the whole specimen leads to an increased detection rate of dysplastic and malignant lesions [52,53]. When this is not the case, the potential for clinically significant lesions to be undetected is increased. It has also been shown that up to 30% of breast resections in which microcalcifications were the mammographic indicator of carcinoma, these calcifications were histologically identified only in benign tissue proximate to the lesion rather than within the malignant structures [54-58]. Such microcalcifications were found in or adjacent to abnormal lobules even in lobular carcinoma *in-situ* [59]. Two studies have shown that the number of paraffin blocks required to sample a whole specimen can vary from 13 [60] to at least 30-40 per case [61]. This would involve an enormous amount of work on the part of those participating in preparation and diagnosis.

A cost-effective method for sampling grossly benign biopsies was presented by Schnitt and Wang [53]. It consists in submitting initially a maximum of 10 blocks of fibrous parenchyma for each case. The remaining tissue is histologically examined only if carcinoma or atypical hyperplasia was found. However, routinely submitting a predetermined number of blocks regardless of specimen size or nature of the mammographic abnormality may be cost effective in terms of reducing the technical work load, but will certainly result in cases of premalignant or malignant lesions being overlooked. It seems, therefore, that it is a practical impossibility to find an ideal method of sampling which can be applied to all kinds of surgical specimens. A possible answer would be to aim for the highest possible yield of pathological abnormalities within the resources available in a routine pathology laboratory. Such a strategy has been followed in our department during the last 10 years by using the large section technique.

The Large Section Technique

Before and after the introduction of screening, an average of 3 to 7 blocks were taken from each breast specimen, but it soon became evident that these small tissue blocks were inadequate for the proper and detailed reporting of mammographically-detected lesions.

A qualitative change was needed. Large paraffin sections were introduced in 1983 and have been used in our department ever since - 43 in 1983 rose to 264 in 1991 representing 10.6% and 63.3%, respectively, of the total number of breast specimens (Fig. 2).

The choice between conventional small and large section techniques depends on the size of the specimen and the nature of the lesion as on mammographic and/or macroscopic examination. Whole lumpectomy, or segment preparations as well as suspicious areas in mastectomies can be examined by this method. An area as big as 10 x 8 cm prepared as a single large section would have needed at least 20 conventional (2 x 2 cm) blocks to assess the same amount of tissue. Using large sections also saves the pathologist the trouble of having to number blocks and then re-assemble them mentally; in terms of time spent by the technician, this means he has to prepare only 1 as opposed to some 20 sections.

When dealing with palpable tumours, the selected slices should show the largest dimension of the mass and the shortest distance to the nearest margin of excision. Should this not be possible in 1 slice, more slices should be taken. The thickness of individual slices should not exceed 0.5 cm. With impalpable lesions, the selection of the proper slices is determined by the mammographic images. The pathologist should be able to project the mammographic image into a histological section, which should include the largest dimension of any abnormality as seen on the mammogram. It is possible, if necessary, to embed the whole specimen in such a way that all excision margins can be assessed without resorting to inking or any other way of marking the surface of the excised tissue. This can involve up to 6 large slices.

Time was the main disadvantage involved in this method. This has now been overcome by a method which has reduced this time to 4 working days. Tissue slices stretched and pinned out on perforated cork are fixed in 10% neutral buffered formalin for 24 hours. They are processed by standard machines according to the following scheme: 70% alcohol for 1.5 hours, 95% alcohol for 18 hours, 3 changes of absolute alcohol totalling 9 hours, 2 changes of xylene totalling 5 hours, and 2 baths of paraffin wax totalling 12 hours. The slices are embedded in "L" shaped pieces approximately 5 cm deep. Wax should cool slowly until a good crust is formed, about the same thickness as the tissue slice. Running water is used to complete the cooling process of the block. Cooling too fast means that the face of the block can shrink. If this happens, melt the block out and re-embed. The blocks are placed in the fridge for 1 hour before cutting. For microtomy we use a Jung (Leica) Polycut, fully automatic machine. However, a heavy duty conventional sledge microtome can produce equally good sections [62]. The sections are stained using an automatic staining machine.

Microwaving Breast Tissue

The use of a microwave oven, however, can substantially reduce the time needed for fixing and/or processing tissue slices. Fixation can be reduced from 24 hours to less than 2 hours and if the whole process is done in the microwave oven, blocks can be produced from fresh tissue in less than 4 hours. The fixative used is "Kryofix" (Merk), which contains a mixture of polyethylene glycol 300, alcohol and distilled water. Further fixation and dehydration is achieved by absolute alcohol. Isopropanol is then used to complete dehydration and to clear the tissue. Impregnation in paraffin wax is even done in the microwave oven. Our laboratory uses a Polaron H2500 microwave oven designed especially for laboratory use by Bio-Rad, Watford, U.K. This type of oven allows control over temperature, time and power level as well as extraction of vapours produced during processing. Resections received in the early hours of a working day can be fixed, processed, sectioned, stained, examined and reported on the same or at most the next working day.

Despite criticism and some misrepresentations (mainly increased costs and "poorer" section quality), large sections are not unique to breast pathology [8,10]. They have been used successfully in diseases other than breast cancer, by neuropathologists, for example, and also in the examination of whole prostates. This method has been adopted since the early 1980s in screening projects in Guildford, U.K., and Falun, Sweden, with a high rate of reproducibility, notwithstanding the different approaches and equipment. All those involved in screening should be trained to meet the requirements of the new situation, and laboratory technicians should not be an exception.

This technique is simple, reproducible, rational and economic. It is inconceivable to screen for breast cancer without using large

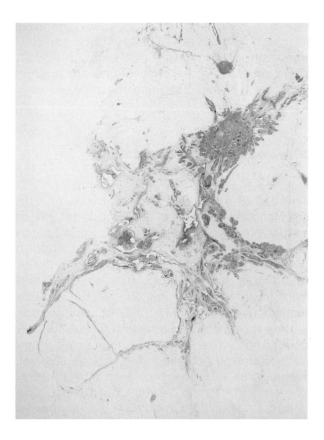

Fig. 3. A 63-year old woman with a tumour shadow and microcalcifications on mammography. A large section showing duct carcinoma *in situ* in an area 4 cm large with 2 infiltrative foci, 3 and 10 mm in diameter. Benign intraductal papillomas are also seen

umenting unsuspected abnormalities, measuring the exact size of the tumour, reporting on multifocality and the state of the resection margins (Fig. 3).

Three-Dimensional Subgross Sampling Technique

This method for the study of the subgross anatomy of breast tissue in animals and humans has been used since 1932 [63]. Recently, it has been modified for use in deprocessed paraffin wax embedded blocks ("Backprocessing") by Jack Davies and Jeanette Armstrong of the Regional Breast Pathology Unit, Southmead Hospital, Bristol, U.K.

The mammographer sees a picture summating the 3-dimensional nature of the lesion in breast tissue. Comparison between pictures provided by mammograms, large histological sections and subgross preparations would be very helpful for educational and research purposes. Subgross preparations reveal the features seen on a mammogram showing the 3-dimensional characteristics of the disease. The complex nature of lesions and their relationship to ducts and terminal ductal-lobular units is shown up (Fig. 4) and together with the large section technique, it can provide information about spatial relationships of early breast disease.

The technique involves dewaxing paraffin blocks and bringing wax-embedded tissues back to water. They are then stained with haematoxylin, differentiated and "blued" as in conventional histology. They are dehydrated in alcohol and cleared with xylene followed by methyl salicylate. The preparations may be viewed in a stereomicroscope after an hour, but improve the longer they are kept in the clearing solution. The thickness range varies from 0.5 to 1.5 mm depending on the type of lesion. Thinner preparations are more suitable for lesions rich in fibroepithelial structures such as sclerosing duct hyperplasia (the so-called radial scar). If necessary, sections of the appropriate thickness are made while the tissues are still soaked in wax after melting the block. Surfaces can be levelled by re-embedding and further trimming using the

sections as they are essential to obtaining optimal information for diagnosis and management of breast cancer. The size of a breast cancer is to be measured on a histological slide and is only determined accurately by microscope. Mammographic or macroscopic measurements of tumour size are to be considered preliminary and not as an alternative to the microscopic size. A full description of the essential characteristics of a cancer is basic information in a histopathological report and should be available in a clear and comprehensive way to the clinician. The nomenclature of breast diseases is far from standardised and such terms as multifocal and multicentric have various connotations when used by different authors. It is also vitally important that the clinician understands the terminology of the pathologist.

Large sections allow mapping of the lesions and studying their spatial relationships, doc-

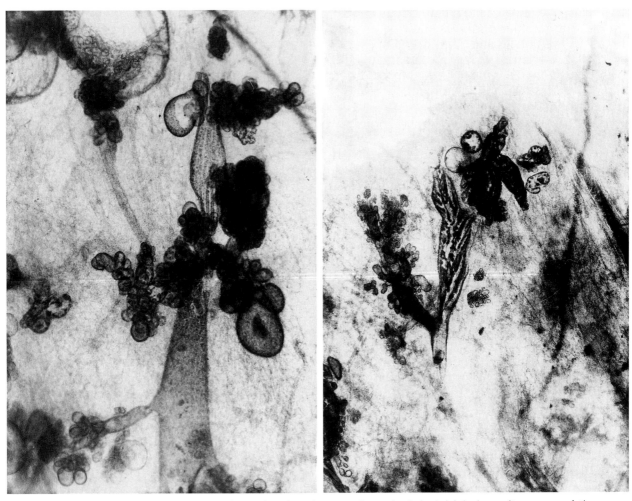

Fig. 4. Subgross 3-dimensional preparations showing ducts and terminal ductal lobular units, some of them are cystically dilated and show microcalcifications. The ducts in the middle of the picture on the right hand side show micropapillary structures. Histologically, this case shows hyperplastic breast disease and micropapillary duct carcinoma *in situ*

microtome. After initial experimentation, this method can be performed in any routine laboratory.

Axillary Dissection Specimen

Lymph nodes are found more readily when the axillary pad of fat is examined unfixed, in the fresh state, by inspection and palpation, whilst slicing the whole preparation. All nodes, irrespective of size, must be processed and examined in toto, large nodes bisected or divided into as many slices as necessary. Bisection in the hilar plane allows for

examination of fewer blocks, whilst revealing metastases with considerable certainty [64].
Clearing agents increase the number of identified lymph nodes as compared with conventional manual dissection [65,66], though their use does not add significant prognostic information [67,68]. This method was used in the Guildford screening programme [62], but was reported by others to be time-consuming and costly in reagents. The use of this method is not regarded as necessary in the search for axillary lymph nodes [8,64].
Our surgeons mark the top of the axillary specimen with a suture and the axilla is then divided randomly into 3 levels. Division is ideally performed if the surgeon has marked the specimen in relation to the margins of the pectoralis minor when dissecting the axilla.

Reporting the state of the lymph nodes should include the number of nodes showing metastases in relation to the total number examined, the presence of micrometastasis, the size of a metastatic node if equal to or larger than 2 cm, as well as the presence of periglandular infiltration.

Quality Assurance and Training

Quality-assurance requirements and objectives have already been laid down and well documented. This author agrees with the principles expressed in the documents issued by the Royal College of Pathologists [7], the cytology subgroup [29] and the Europe Against Cancer programme [69]. Nevertheless, the necessity of adhering to locally agreed guidelines cannot be understressed. A critically determining factor in the outcome of a breast cancer screening programme and, in particular, the reduction of mortality, is the substantial experience in breast pathology, including cytological and histopathological diagnosis of the pathologist.

Every screening centre should include in its multidisciplinary team of mammographer, surgeon and oncologist an expert breast pathologist. Such an expert should have the following responsibilities: to maintain standards of diagnosis and reporting of screened cases, the documentation of lesions, the teaching of colleagues and junior staff, the organisation of local training programmes and quality assurance. Teaching and training should be tailored to the status and experience of said pathologist. Specialists should attend introductory courses at recognised training centres and these centres should be nominated by the experts in the respective countries. The length of the introductory course should be individually assessed, whereas trainee pathologists should be given more comprehensive training in techniques, namely, dissection of breast specimens, selection of blocks and documentation of findings.

Workshops and consultation with the reference pathologist in difficult or doubtful cases are strongly recommended and form the basis for collecting materials for training and quality assurance.

Conclusion

The performance of all the members of the multidisciplinary team should be optimal and the pathologist's role within it is critical in the effort to reduce mortality. In conclusion, the judgement of the pathologist does not only affect the treatment of the patient, but also the mammographer and the selection criteria by way of the "feedback mechanism" initiated by the pathology report. Of greater importance too, especially when rates of over- or underdiagnosis are significant, is an overall muddling of statistics, thereby invalidating any serious attempt to analyse the screening programme overall. This statement was made some 8 years ago [70] and is still valid.

Acknowledgement

I am deeply indebted to the following friends and colleagues:
Dr. Jack Davies and Dr. Jeanette Armstrong for their advice on the subgross 3-dimensional method, Dr. Mathilde Boon of Leiden, the Netherlands, and her technical team for their invaluable contribution to the development of the microwave method, Dr. Clive Wells and Dr. Marigold Curling, of the Department of Cytology, St. Bartholomew's Hospital, London, U.K., for informing me about the British Guidelines on Cytology, and Dr. László Tabár for his valuable discussions. Thanks are due to Hedley Glencross of the Princess Royal Hospital, Haywards Heath, U.K., for expert technical assistance with the microwave and subgross 3-dimensional methods, Kathrin Dahl-Qvist for secretarial assistance, and Gösta Andersson for photography.

REFERENCES

1   Tabár L, Fagerberg G, Duffy SW, Day NE, Gad A, Gröntoft O: Update of the Swedish Two County program of mammographic screening for breast cancer. Radiol Clin N Amer 1992 (30):187-210

2   Azavedo E, Svane G, Ringertz H: The role of the radiologist in screening for nonpalpable breast tumours in Sweden. Invest Radiol 1991 (26):174-178

3   Blamey R: Place and training of the surgeon in breast cancer screening. Aust N Z J Surg 1989 (59):303-306

4   Shapiro S: More on screening and breast cancer incidence. JNCI 1991 (83):1522-1523

5   Elston CW, Ellis IO: Pathology and breast screening. Histo-pathology 1990 (16):109-118

6   Elston CW: The United Kingdom National Breast Screening Programme: implications for pathology departments. Med Lab Sci 1989 (46):223-229

7   Royal College of Pathologists Working Party. Guidelines for Pathologists. Oxford Screening Publications, 1990

8   Royal College of Pathologists Working Party. Pathology Reporting in Breast Cancer Screening. Oxford Screening Publications, 1990

9   Gad A: Screening for breast cancer: examination and reporting of histopathological preparations. Lancet 1988 (ii):953

10 Armstrong JS, Davies JD: Laboratory handling of impalpable breast lesions: A review. J Clin Pathol 1991 (44):89-93

11 Sloane JP: Changing role of the pathologist. Brit Med Bulletin 1991 (47):433-454

12 Schnitt SJ, Connolly JL: Processing and evaluation of breast excision specimens. A clinically oriented approach. Amer J Clin Path 1992 (98):125-137

13 Green B, McDicken IW, Turnbull LS: Implications on laboratory workload of breast cancer screening. J Clin Pathol 1992 (45):521-523

14 Holmberg L, Adami H-O, Persson I, Lundström T, Tabár L: Demands on surgical inpatient services after mass mammographic screening. Br Med J 1986 (293):779-782

15 Tabár L, Gad A, Holmberg L, Ljungquist U: Significant reduction in advanced breast cancer. Results of the first seven years of mammography screening in Kopparberg, Sweden. Diag Imag Clin Med 1985 (54):158-164

16 Kline TS: Survey of aspiration biopsy cytology of breast. Diagn Cytopathol 1991 (7):98-105

17 Franzén S, Zajicek J: Aspiration biopsy in diagnosis of palpable lesions of the breast: Critical review of 3479 consecutive biopsies. Acta Radiol 1968 (7):241-262

18 Zajdela A, Chossein NA, Pillerton JP: The value of aspiration cytology in the diagnosis of breast cancer. Cancer 1975 (35):499-506

19 Masood S, Frykberg ER, McLellan GL, Scalapino MC, Mitchum DG, Bullard JB: Prospective evaluation of radiologically directed fine needle aspiration biopsy of nonpalpable breast lesions. Cancer 1990 (66):1480-1487

20 Fornage BD: Percutaneous biopsies of the breast: State of the art. Cardiovasc Intervent Radiol 1991 (14):29-39

21 Jewell WR, Thomas J, Chang CHJ: Computed tomographic mammography directed biopsy of the breast. Surg Gynecol Obstet 1983 (157):75-76

22 Giard RW, Hermans J: The value of aspiration cytologic examination of the breast. A statistical review of the medical literature. Cancer 1992 (69):2104-2110

23 Fagerberg G, Mansson JC: Directional aspiration biopsy under mammographic guidance. Path Biol 1991 (39):847

24 Löfgren M, Andersson I, Bondeson L, Lindholm K: X-ray guided fine-needle aspiration for the cytologic diagnosis of non-palpable breast lesions. Cancer 1988 (61):1032-1037

25 Svane G, Silfverswärd C: Stereotaxic needle biopsy of nonpalpable breast lesions. Acta Radiol Diag 1983 (24):283-288

26 Azavedo E, Svane G, Auer G: Stereotactic fine needle biopsy in 2594 mammographically detected non-palpable lesions. Lancet 1989 (i):1033-1036

27 Ciatto S, Rosselli Del Turco M, Bravetti P: Nonpalpable breast lesions: Stereotaxic fine-needle aspiration cytology. Radiol 1989 (173):57-59

28 Graham IH: Fine-needle biopsy in mammographically detected non-palpable lesions. Letter to the Editor. Lancet 1989 (ii):384

29 Cytology Subgroup of the National Co-ordinating Committee for Breast Cancer Screening Pathology. Guidelines for Cytology Procedures and Reporting in Breast Cancer Screening. NHSBSP Screening Publications, London September 1992

30 Swedish National Board of Health and Welfare. Mammographic Screening for Breast Cancer. Cytopathology Guidelines. (in press)

31 Frisell J, Eklund G, Nilsson R, Hellström L, Somell A: Additional value of fine-needle aspiration biopsy in a mammographic screening trial. Br J Surg 1989 (76):840-843

32 Ciatto S: Usefulness of needle aspiration in a screening programme. In: Ziant G (ed) Practical Modalities of an Efficient Screening for Breast

Cancer in the European Community. Elsevier Science Publisher B.U., 1989 pp 83-84

33 Parker SH, Lovin JD, Jobe WE: Stereotactic breast biopsy with a biopsy gun. Radiol 1990 (176):741-747

34 Parker SH, Lovin JD, Jobe WE, Burke BJ, Hopper KD, Yakes WF: Nonpalpable breast lesions: Stereotactic automated large core biopsies. Radiol 1991 (180):403-407

35 Dronkers DJ: Stereotaxic core biopsy of breast lesions. Radiol 1992 (183):631-634

36 Dowlatshahi K, Gent JG, Schmidt R, Jokich PM, Bibbo M, Sprenger E: Nonpalpable breast tumours: diagnosis with stereotaxic localization and fine-needle aspiration. Radiol 1989 (170):427-433

37 Svane G: A stereotaxic technique for preoperative marking of nonpalpable breast lesions. Acta Radiol 1983 (24):145-151

38 Frank HA, Hall FM, Steer ML: Preoperative localization of non-palpable breast lesions demonstrated by mammography. New Engl J Med 1976 (295):259-260

39 Snyder RE: Specimen radiography and preoperative localization of non-palpable breast cancer. Cancer 1980 (46):950-956

40 Holland R: The role of specimen X-ray in the diagnosis of breast cancer. Diag Imag Clin Med 1985 (54):178-185

41 Wilkinson EJ, Gnadt JT, Milbrath J, Clowry LJ: Breast biopsy evaluation by paraffin-block radiography. Arch Pathol Lab Med 1978 (102):470-473

42 Snyder RE, Rosen P: Radiography of breast specimens. Cancer 1971 (28):1608-1611

43 Rosen PP: Frozen section diagnosis of breast lesions. Recent experience with 556 consecutive biopsies. Am Surg 1978 (187):17-19

44 Zarbo RJ, Hoffman GG, Howanitz PJ: Interinstitutional comparison of frozen-section consultation. A college of American pathologists Q-probe study of 79 647 consultations in 297 North American Institutions. Arch Pathol Lab Med 1991 (115):1187-1194

45 Oberman HA: A modest proposal. Am J Surg Pathol (16):69-70

46 Anderson TJ: The pathologist and breast cancer screening. J Pathol 1987 (153):309-312

47 Anonymous: Back-up for screening for breast cancer. Br M J 1978 (277):153-154

48 Fisher B: Reappraisal of breast biopsy prompted by the use of lumpectomy. Surgical strategy. JAMA 1985 (253):3585-3588

49 Holmberg L, Tabár L, Gad A: Treatment of breast cancer detected on screening in Sweden. In: Feig SA, McLelland R (eds) Breast Carcinoma, Current

Diagnosis and Treatment. Masson Publishing, USA 1983 pp 627-631

50 Aspgren K, Holmberg L, Adami H-O: Standardization of the surgical technique in breast conserving treatment of mammography cancer. Br J Surg 1988 (75):807-810

51 Leis Jr HP: Breast biopsy: Indications and techniques. Breast, Diseases of the breast 1980 (6):2-6

52 Patchefsky AS, Potok J, Hoch WS, Libshitz HI: Increased detection of occult breast carcinoma after more thorough histologic examination of breast biopsies. Am J Clin Pathol 1973 (60):799-804

53 Schnitt SJ, Wang HH: Histologic sampling of grossly benign breast biopsies: How much is enough? Am J Surg Pathol 1989 (13):505-512

54 Price JL, Gibbs NM: The relationship between microcalcification and in situ carcinoma of the breast. Clin Radiol 1978 (29):447-452

55 Murphy WA, Deschryver-Kecskemeti K: Isolated clustered microcalcifications in the breast: Radiologic-pathologic correlation. Radiol 1978 (127):335-341

56 Roses DF, Harris MN, Gorstein F, Gumport SL: Biopsy for microcalcification detected by mammography. Surgery 1980 (87):248-252

57 Colbassani HJ, Feller WF, Cigtay OS, Chun B: Mammographic and pathologic correlation of microcalcification in disease of breast. Surg Gynecol Obstet 1982 (155):689-696

58 Prorok JJ, Trostle DR, Scarlato M, Rachman R: Excisional breast biopsy and roentgenographic examination for mammographically detected microcalcification. Am J Surg 1983 (145):684-686

59 Snyder RE: Mammography and lobular carcinoma in-situ. Surg Gynecol Obstet 1966 (122):255-260

60 Schnitt SJ, Wang HH, Owings DV, Hann L: Sampling grossly benign breast biopsy specimens. Lancet 1989 (ii):1038

61 Gallager HS: Breast specimen radiography. Obligatory adjuvant and investigative. Am J Clin Pathol 1975 (64):749-755

62 Gibbs N: Large paraffin sections and chemical clearance of axillary tissues as a routine procedure in the pathological examination of the breast. Histopathol 1982 (6):647-660

63 Sarnelli R, Sabb C, Squartini F: Subgross physiopathology of the breast associated with clinical cancer. Tumori 1980 (66):565-582

64 Hartveit F: The routine histological investigation of axillary lymph nodes for metastatic breast cancer. J Pathol 1984 (143):187-191

65 Fisher B, Slack N: Number of nodes examined in the prognosis of breast carcinoma. Surg Gynecol

Obstet 1970 (131):79-88

66 Durkin K, Haagenesen CD: An improved technique for the study of lymph nodes in surgical specimens. Ann Surg 1980 (191):419-429

67 Morrow M, Evans J, Rosen PP, Kinne DW: Does clearing of axillary lymph nodes contribute to accurate staging of breast carcinoma? Cancer 1984 (53):1329-1332

68 Kingsley WB, Peters GN, Cheek H: What constitutes adequate study of axillary lymph nodes in breast cancer? Ann Surg 1985 (201):311-314

69 Europe Against Cancer. European Guidelines for Quality Assurance in Mammography Screening. Document DGV-775-92, May 1992

70 Gad A, Thomas BA, Moskowitz M (eds) Screening for Breast Cancer in Europe: Achievements, Problems, and Future. Recent Results in Cancer Research. Springer-Verlag Berlin, Heidelberg 1984 pp 179-194

Therapeutic Aspects of Screen-Detected Lesions: The Role of the Surgeon

Roger Blamey

Nottingham City Hospital, Hucknall Road, Nottingham NG5 1PB, United Kingdom

Screening detects breast cancers at a small and curable size. To take full advantage of this, the detected tumours must be treated optimally. There is no single treatment suitable for all primary breast cancers as they present with different characteristics which need different types of management. Criteria may now be set out to guide treatment; some based on good evidence and testing, some on what are at present theoretically derived protocols which are being tested in trials.

The Need for Specialisation

An understanding of these management criteria requires a surgeon with a special interest in breast cancer. The criteria on which cancer management decisions are based include histopathological and radiological characteristics. The management of screen-detected tumours has become a team effort: the surgeon may expect breast cancer expertise on the part of his pathological and radiological colleagues; similarly, they may expect to work with a surgeon who has acquired such expertise, i.e. a surgeon who attends assessment clinics, takes part in diagnostic decisions, carries out the steriotactic marker biopsies and treats cancer cases in accordance with the team's protocols.

Many units within the U.K. now have such teams and, as a result, screen-detected breast cancers receive treatment by a specialised team. However, cancers presenting outside the screening programme do not receive such attention. It is the contention of the author (and the way in which work is carried out in the Nottingham City Hospital unit) that the team which has gained the necessary expertise should look after the symptomatically presenting breast cancers, in addition to the screen-detected. In other words, there has to be specialisation, with a surgeon taking breast cancer as a main interest (in smaller hospitals perhaps combining this with a second speciality such as colon cancer). Such specialisation is the general drift from general surgery, with urology, thoracic and vascular surgery and upper GI endoscopy already largely specialised. In the same way radiology has introduced specialist interest among consultants, and pathology is following.

Standards

In the care of breast disease, the introduction of screening has led to the recognition that special expertise is required. In the U.K., this has resulted in the publication of documents on standards in radiography, radiology, surgery and pathology.

Expected Standards of Surgery in Breast Cancer Screening

The responsibility for surgical audit lies with the Royal Colleges of Surgery. At the commencement of breast cancer screening, a group of interested surgeons was formed within the British Association of Surgical Oncology (BASO). This group was asked to set up a formal structure linking with the National Coordinator for Breast Cancer

Screening (then Dr. Muir Grey) and referred to, for short, as the BASO Group. One surgical co-ordinator per health region (covering a total population of 3-4 million people) liaises with the central and regional initiatives and with the other surgeons participating in screening in their region. A total of 190 surgeons take part in breast cancer screening and perhaps less than half of these might be described as having specialist expertise in breast disease.

The aims of the surgical group were expressed in the report of a working party of the Royal College of Surgeons under the chairmanship of Professor Patrick Boulter:

That the Surgical Colleges should take an active training and monitoring role in breast cancer screening; that screening centres should have appointed surgical input to participate in clinical assessment and carry out the necessary surgical procedures and that the surgeon should be part of a multidisciplinary team.

The BASO group drew up "Quality Assurance Guidelines for Surgeons in Breast Screening". This document was approved by the Royal Colleges of Surgeons and has now been published by Dr. Joan Austoker as an NHS Breast Screening Publication [1].

In addition to issuing the Guidelines, the BASO group meets regularly and has certain other duties. The group has 30 members and each health service region, the Royal Surgical Colleges, the main BASO organisation, and Colleges of Radiology and Pathology are represented on it.

Quality Assurance (QA)

Each regional surgical coordinator is responsible for arranging an annual meeting in his/her region of surgeons who are engaged in breast cancer screening. One surgeon has been identified per screening unit to present the surgical audit data at the annual meeting; the ability of each unit to adhere to the Guidelines may then be assessed. Some health regions have organised quality assurance visits to their units and the regional surgical coordinator, who is a member of the Regional screening QA committee, nominates the visiting surgeon for these visits.

Training

The BASO group is presenting suggestions to the Royal Colleges of Surgeons for the training of surgeons who will take part in screening. It is recognised that screening is only a part of breast cancer care. Some surgeons intend to take a specialised role in breast disease in a major centre, while others wish to become a surgeon at a breast clinic and be involved in breast cancer screening in a smaller, district general hospital.

The BASO group suggests that surgeons applying for such posts should have spent, during the higher surgical training, a year in a recognised major unit. A tentative list of such units has been drawn up, using the criteria that a major unit should have: a high patient throughput from the symptomatic clinics, screening, a significant research output, access to reconstructive surgery. Before that, during their registrar period of training, they should have spent 6 months on a firm of 2 consultants, one of whom has a special interest in breast disease and is engaged in screening work. Such posts would be largely in district general hospitals and a list of suggested surgeons with such an interest is being compiled.

A multidisciplinary course on breast screening is held in Nottingham and this includes a surgical section. There are also update courses organised at this centre on specific topics in breast screening surgery, e.g., the management of DCIS.

Education

The BASO group holds regular workshop sessions on aspects of surgery related to breast cancer screening, such as the management of patients with risk factors, the management of small, very good prognosis tumours and surgical techniques in screening.

The Guidelines for Surgeons [1]

The published guidelines make many clinical recommendations and set certain standards.

Attendance at Assessment/Recall

The guidelines state that the surgeon should be available to see patients in the re-call/assessment clinics. The surgeon does not need to examine all cases brought back for assessment, e.g., those simply recalled for an extra mammographic view which then rules out the presence of a radiological abnormality. The surgeon must be able to examine the breast prior to any invasive diagnostic procedure (FNAC or needle biopsy); if not, he may be faced with a woman with a palpable lump in the breast, which may or may not have undergone a considerable change in clinical signs and size due to bruising from the needle procedure. It is impossible to make decisions on diagnostic excision or on cancer management in such a situation.

Guidelines Helpful to the Surgeon

The surgeon forms part of a multidisciplinary team and may expect expertise from pathologists and radiologists. He should have a good cytology service, receive accurate pathological information on benign lesions (including comment on any atypia), on carcinomas *in situ* and on invasive tumours (including grading, typing and sampling of the excision margins). The surgeon may expect to be aided by extremely accurate wire placement for needle localisation biopsies.

A woman awaiting surgical diagnostic biopsy or treatment of a diagnosed breast cancer should not be faced with the anxiety of a long wait. The surgeon must be put into the position of being able to treat the cases as they arise in the programme and not have to build up a waiting list. The standard is that 90% of operations should be carried out within 21 days of the surgical decision to operate.

The surgeon should have the help of a breast care nurse in counselling the patients.

Standards for the Surgeon to Observe

The surgeon and his/her colleagues must attempt to get a preoperative microscopical diagnosis of cancer, and at least 60% of screen-detected cancers should have such a preoperative diagnosis.

An open biopsy required for diagnostic reasons must be carried out with a view to giving a good cosmetic result, since the lesion may prove benign. The standards are that more than 95% of impalpable lesions should be correctly identified at the first marker-wire-localisation operation and that 80% of biopsies which prove benign should weigh < 20 g (weight of the biopsy is the only convenient measure of a likely cosmetic result).

All surgeons involved in the treatment of screen-detected cancers must be aware that different treatment options are available. Every woman should receive information on treatment options and, where appropriate, be offered one of these options. The Guidelines suggest that more than 50% of women with invasive tumours ≤ 15 mm should receive conservative treatment.

Specimens must so taken for the pathological examination of margins. The node status of invasive tumours should be determined. Prophylactic axillary irradiation is inappropriate for well-differentiated, node-negative cases, as it is for DCIS. Local excision is inappropriate for extensive DCIS.

Effects on Symptomatic Breast Work

The standards illustrated above have resulted in a general increase in the levels of surgical expertise in the care of breast cancer. Similar improvements in expertise in radiography, mammographic radiology, histology and fine-needle aspiration cytology of the breast have followed.

There are also some specific effects on practice in symptomatically presenting breast problems. For example, it has been the practice for benign feeling solid breast lumps to be excised for a full diagnosis. In screening, similar but impalpable lesions are seen, and if the radiologist judges them as benign, then they are left *in situ*. We are thus confronted with a paradox: a palpable lump that can be felt and seems benign on FNAC is removed; whereas the impalpable lump, which cannot be palpated and on which no FNAC is performed, is left *in situ*. For this reason, in Nottingham we now have a diagnostic proto-

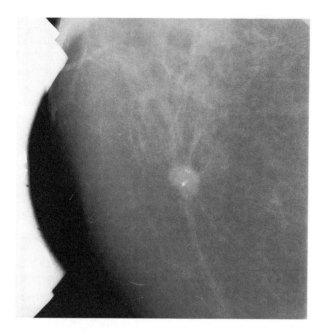

Fig. 1. A spiculate lesion, radiologically rated as a suspect carcinoma: on marker localisation, biopsy proved to be a radial scar

col using imaging and FNAC to prove that a benign-feeling lump is in fact benign and thus save the patient from an operation. The multidisciplinary approach applies to all breast problems, whether from screening or with symptoms.

Marker-Wire Localisation Biopsy

Operation with marker localisation may be carried out for therapeutic reasons when there is a preoperative cytological diagnosis of cancer, or for diagnostic reasons when there is not. The former requires a wide excision around the marked centre of the lesion: the cancer can often be felt between the fingers after superficial subcutaneous dissection and deep dissection on the pectoral fascia. Nevertheless, accurate marking is very important to the surgeon. A specimen X-ray should be taken to ensure that the cancer is taken with sufficient margins all round.

When operating for diagnostic reasons, it has to be remembered that the lesion may be benign. Therefore, a good cosmetic result should be aimed at obtaining a small scar

right over the lesion with as small a piece of tissue as possible removed [2]. Good marking and a marker wire set which has a cannula to slide over the wire, in order that the surgeon may easily feel the tip and incise directly over it, e.g., the "Nottingham Needle" (Mediplus U.K. Ltd), are required. The Guidelines suggest that pieces of less than 20 g should be removed - our own median is 8 g (Fig. 2).

Excised Benign Lesions

An excised benign lesion is, in retrospect, a surgical error. A woman has been frightened into believing she may well have cancer and has had to undergo an operation she did not need. The radiological features of some lesions (or sometimes the clinical findings) are such that the possibility of cancer is high and they have to be excised for histological examination (Fig. 1). The histologies of benign lesions excised in the prevalence round of the Nottingham programme are shown in Table 1.

Benign lesions are most often excised in the prevalence round of screening: they have been present in the breast for many years and there are no previous films allowing for a comparison of possible progression. The Surgical Guidelines state that no more than 9 benign lesions per 1,000 women screened should be excised and that the ratio of cancers detected in the programme to benign lesions excised should be 1:1; in fact, several units in the U.K. are achieving ratios of 3 cancers diagnosed to 1 benign lesion excised in the prevalence round.

Table 1. Benign lesions excised from screening 30,000 women

Fibrocystic change/nor	45
Fibroadenoma	27
Radial scar	21
Sclerosing adenosis	9
Papilloma	3
Atypical ductal hyperplasia	1
	____
	106

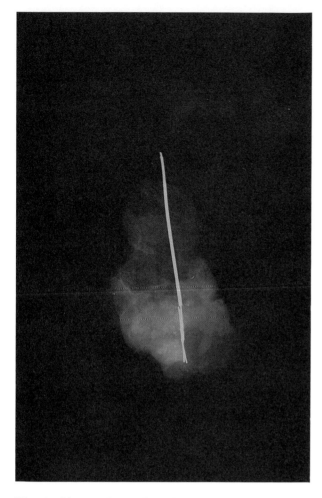

Fig. 2. Diagnostic marker-wire biopsy. The piece of tissue removed weighed 6 g and the lesion is clearly seen

The avoidance of benign biopsy depends on radiological expertise and experience, and is aided considerably by fine-needle aspiration cytology of impalpable lesions. In Nottingham over 80% of impalpable cancers are diagnosed preoperatively by ultrasound- or stereo-guided cytology. This level of sensitivity for cancer diagnosis increases confidence in the use of cytology to help establish that a lesion is benign.

Cancers Detected at Screening

DCIS

Around 17% of cancers detected in the prevalence round of screening are DCIS. The out-come of DCIS treated by mastectomy is very good, with few deaths from breast cancer and no local recurrences over the succeeding years [3]. Conservative treatment - with or without breast irradiation - carries a high rate of local recurrence. Holland [4] has demonstrated that DCIS is frequently extensive. Since recurrence usually occurs at the site of excision, it seems likely that incompleteness of excision is the cause of local recurrence.

Our own practice is to carry out mastectomy (or subcutaneous mastectomy) if radiology indicates that the disease is extensive (> 3-4 cm). If the disease appears localised on mammography, then wide excision is performed, with re-excision of any margin with less than 5 mm of clear tissue. Breast irradiation is not given. If the pathology shows extensive DCIS, conversion to mastectomy is undertaken.

In the U.K., there are 2 clinical studies in DCIS. The UKCCCR trial examines recurrence in the breast after complete excision (CE) of localised DCIS with the following 4 arms: CE only, CE + irradiation (RT), CE + tamoxifen, and CE + RT + tamoxifen.

The BASO I registration study examines occurrence of contralateral breast cancer after treatment of DCIS by mastectomy. The arms are no added treatment or tamoxifen for 5 years.

Invasive Cancers with Excellent Prognosis

The Nottingham prognostic index is a prospectively confirmed index, which gives powerful survival predictions for any patient [5]. The index is based on histological grade, lymph-node stage and tumour size. A patient with a grade I tumour (well differentiated), lymph-node negative and 2 cm or less in diameter, has a survival chance at 15 years equivalent to that of a woman who does not have breast cancer (Fig. 3). This group of tumours may be considered cured and, as seen in Table 2, accounts for around 40% of tumours detected at screening. These tumours are often tubular mixed, tubular or cribriform; unlike DCIS (to which they have a similar prognosis), they are often not extensive within the breast.

Our method of management is to achieve

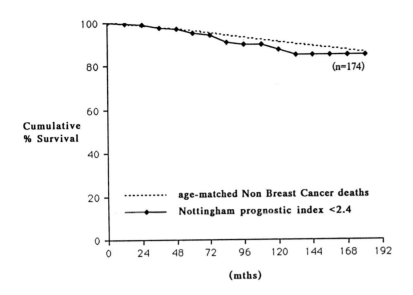

Fig. 3. Survival curves of women with tumours of Nottingham Prognostic Index ≤ 2.4 (grade I, LN negative, ≤ 2 cm) compared with survival of age-matched female population without breast cancer

histologically confirmed complete excision and to withhold breast irradiation. We do not surgically clear nor irradiate the axillary nodes, since there is little or no chance of symptomatic nodal recurrence in the follow-up. We do not give adjuvant systemic therapy since these patients may be considered cured by their primary surgery and have no metastases to be treated with systemic therapy. We have treated around 52 similar lesions in this way in the past 2 years. Follow-up is very short but we have no recurrences to report, neither local nor metastatic.

There is a multicentre trial (BASO II) established in the U.K. for the treatment of well-differentiated grade I or special type, lymph-node negative, small primary tumours. The arms are complete excision only, CE + RT, CE + tamoxifen and CE + RT + tamoxifen.

Higher grade or larger tumours detected at screening are treated according to our usual protocols for symptomatically presenting breast cancers.

Table 2. Cancers detected in the prevalence round of screening (30,000 women screened)

DCIS	34
LCIS	NIL
Invasive	149
Grade 1, LN negative, ≤ 2 cm 60	
Intermediate prognosis 81	
Locally advanced 8	

Summary

The main intention behind the introduction of breast cancer screening in the UK was to reduce the death rate from breast cancer. However, there are other beneficial effects; more tumours are likely to be suitable for breast conservation. Perhaps the major effect has been the improvement in the services for women with breast disease: a high-quality service for patients from the screening programme is translated through to the women presenting symptomatically. There are of course some harmful effects from screening - unnecessary biopsies on benign disease and the cosmetic effects of these. In all these aspects, the surgeon plays a major role. A BASO group of surgeons who have breast cancer as their major interest has been formed in the UK. Women suffering from breast cancer are increasingly able to turn to surgeons specialising in the care of their disease. The majority of cancers detected at screening have an excellent prognosis. Localised DCIS is treated by CE alone; the need for RT or tamoxifen to be added is being tested in a clinical trial. Extensive DCIS requires mastectomy. Small invasive tumours may often be treated with breast conservation and, when well differentiated, probably do not need intact breast irradiation and certainly do not require adjuvant systemic therapy.

REFERENCES

1   Quality Assurance Guidelines for Surgeons in Breast Cancer Screening. NHS BSP publication, Sheffield May 1992
2   Blamey RW: Operations for benign conditions of the breast: indications and techniques. In: Smallwood and Taylor (eds) Benign Breast Disease. Edward Arnold, London 1989 pp 142-154
3   Schnitt SJ, Silen W, Sadowsky NL, Connolly JL, Harris JR: Ductal carcinoma in situ (intraductal carcinoma) of the breast. N Engl J Med 1988 (318):898
4   Holland R, Hendriks JHCL, Verbeek ALM, Mravunac M, Schurrmans Stekhoven JH: Extent, distribution, and mammographic/histological correlations of breast ductal carcinoma in situ. Lancet 1990 (335):519-522
5   Gales MH, Blamey RW, Elston CW, Ellis TO: The Nottingham Prognostic Index in primary breast cancer. Breast Cancer Research & Treatment 1992 (22):207-219

Monitoring the Impact of a Breast Cancer Screening Programme

Eugenio Paci [1] and Nicholas E. Day [2]

1 Epidemiology Unit, Centro per lo Studio e la Prevenzione Oncologica, Viale A. Volta 171, 50131 Florence, Italy
2 Medical Research Council, Biostatistic Unit, Shaftesbury Road, Cambridge CB2 2BW, United Kingdom

Several experimental and non-experimental studies support the conclusion that mammographic screening is an effective tool in rc ducing breast cancer mortality in women older than 50 [1]. On the basis of the evidence of efficacy, screening programmes have been started or planned at national or regional level in Europe.

Mortality reduction is the main endpoint of a screening programme, but several years will be required (8-10 according to the experience of the trials) to achieve and estimate evidence of the efficacy of the programme in the population. Early indicators of the screening process are necessary for an early evaluation of the impact of screening. Monitoring of the process is especially important also because the performance of a screening programme is generally expected to be lower than that observed in controlled studies.

Today the results of several programmes assessed by follow-up or case-control studies are available for an estimate of early indicators of efficacy. In particular, recently published data of the W-E trial [2] will be useful to provide a referential exemplification of the screening rationale. On the basis of the W-E trial results, Day et al. [3] proposed some main criteria for monitoring the screening process and this framework will be followed in this paper.

The collection of a minimum set of data should be planned in service screening prior to the implementation of the programme and the whole screening process should be considered starting with the lists of the target population up to the follow-up of the breast cancer cases to assess deaths from breast cancer. The process should also be monitored for the evaluation of the test performance, the diagnostic work-up and the treatment modalities.

Rationale of the Screening Process

Since the efficacy of mammography has been proved in several studies, the relationship between the reduction of mortality and the stage shift of breast cancer can be assessed. The screening test picks up cancers at an earlier stage and the diagnostic modality (screen detected vs clinically detected) and the pathologic classification of the case are related to the lead-time distribution, i.e., are indicators of the diagnostic anticipation. The outcome of screening is due to the success of the treatment of early cancer in producing a better prognosis. In Figures 1 and 2, the cumulative rates of advanced carcinomas and breast cancer mortality in the W-E trial are presented by years from randomisation. A temporal relationship between the 2 reductions is evident, strongly suggesting that the decreasing rate of advanced carcinomas might be the best way to assess the reduction of mortality which will be achieved after a few years.

Recently published data by Duffy et al. [4] and the update of the W-E trial results allow for a more detailed study of the 3 most important prognostic factors for the prediction of the impact of screening: tumour size, nodal status and pathological grade of malignancy. Modification of the prognostic factors depends on early diagnosis by screening and induces a better survival of cancers detected at the screening test. Cancers clinically diag-

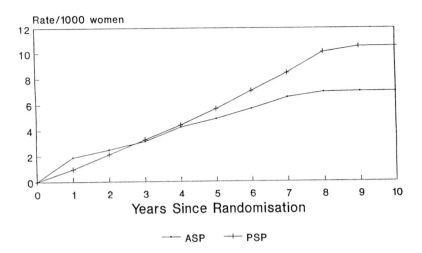

Fig. 1. Cumulative rate of Stage II + cancer, Swedish WE trial. Control (PSP) and Study group (ASP) [2]

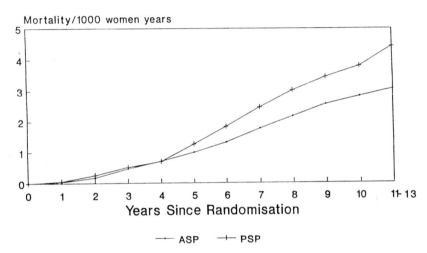

Fig. 2. Cumulative mortality of breast cancer. Swedish WE trial. Control (PSP) and Study group (ASP) [2]

nosed in non-attendant women or in women who have had a negative test (interval cancers) are failures of the screening programme and reduce the impact. Neither of the last 2 categories experience any lead time, showing a stage distribution similar (or worse) to that observed in control groups or in a comparable population.

Background Information

In service screening a comparable control group would not be available because in the future it will be neither ethical nor possible to exclude women from the invitation to take a mammogram. In the Malmö trial, Andersson has shown that in the control group too, 28% of the women had a preventive mammogram outside the screening programme [5].

A comparison of the service performance with that expected in the absence of screening is available from 2 sources. Firstly, from the experience of a similar but still unscreened population, usually a contiguous geographic area; secondly, from the knowledge of the historical experience of breast cancer care in the catchment population. Mortality and incidence rates, by 5-year age group, should be estimated for the period preceding the screening programme. Descriptive epidemiological surveys will provide information on staging and on the diagnostic and treatment practices in the area. For example, an epidemiological description of the use of breast conserving surgery and radiotherapy in the catchment population might be of great interest.

The existence of a tumour registry, recording all cancer cases in a population, is fundamental to the evaluation, but, if not available, a pathology registry of breast cancer incident cases and mortality should be established.

Process Indicators

Participation in the Programme

Breast cancer screening is usually organised in Europe as a public health service and women are personally invited to have a free mammogram every 2-3 years. The participation rate in the programme is a strong predictor of its impact. In fact, cases occurring in non-attenders are clinically diagnosed, usually with a worse staging, and they could have a higher mortality rate than cases in a comparable population. Low compliance to the invitation is detrimental not only to programme efficacy, but also because women not participating might be a group at a higher risk of dying from the disease and/or members of the population with fewer opportunities of using the public services. Lists of the target population should be accurate, including as eligible women the socially weaker groups such as migrants. Where cooperation with general practitioners is possible, it is important to check the lists and ascertain the overall status of the woman concerned, her condition of health (previous breast cancer, terminal illness or psychiatric diseases) and the assessment of her attitude towards screening. Inequalities in access to screening need to be evaluated and corrected by way of informed promotion of participation; this means the discussion of fears and prejudices and also the respect of culturally-based refusals [6].

The compliance rate will be estimated by 5-year age group and possibly by socio-demographic characteristics. An evaluation of the satisfaction of those participating and of the factors determining non-attendance should be carried out by periodic surveys [7].

Test Performance

The main objective of the screening test is to pick up early breast cancers and the detection rate (DR) is the ratio between the number of cancers detected at screening and the number of screened women (usually expressed per 1,000 women screened).

The rate at the first screening depends on the sensitivity of the test and on the mean sojourn time in the so-called detectable preclinical phase [8,9]. At the first screening test, when a population in steady state is screened, it is usual to quote this rate as a "prevalence rate". At the subsequent screenings, cancers with a longer preclinical duration should have been picked up and only new cancers with a shorter preclinical duration will be detected. It is usual to speak of an "incidence rate" at the subsequent screenings and the measure of the detection rate is expected to be lower. The DR increases with age because the preclinical and clinical incidences increase with age and also because mammography has a higher sensitivity at older ages. The DR at the first and repeated screening tests should be presented by 5-year age groups.

To know the programme performance, the detection rate at first and repeated screening tests should be compared to the expected incidence in the screened population in the absence of screening and presented, by age, as a prevalence/incidence ratio (P/I) [10]. Table 1 shows the measures of DR and P/I in the main programmes already published [11]. The expected incidence rate in the screened women would be estimated from the incidence rate in the total population, adjusting for the proportion of attendance and the rate of incidence in non-attenders, according to the following identity [3]:

incidence rate in the total population = P x incidence rate in attenders +(1-P) x incidence rate in refusers

where P is the real compliance rate (expressed as proportion). The correction might be relevant if the selection of screened women is important and the estimate is not adjusted for the determinants of the risk of dying from breast cancer which might have determined the selection.

Stage Distribution of Screen-Detected Cancer

The screening impact depends on the ability of the test to detect cancers earlier and the W-

Table 1. Prevalence rates seen at the first screening round in the HIP, Utrecht and Swedish studies and in the Florence district programme

Study	Age group	Number of cases	Prevalence x 1,000 women screened	Prevalence rate/annual incidence rate
HIP	40-64	55	2.93	1.30
Sweden	40-49	40	2.15	1.95
	50-59	101	4.63	3.09
	60-69	190	9.08	4.59
Utrecht	50-59	63	6.20	2.95
	60-64	43	9.51	3.80
Florence district	40-44	7	0.78	0.76
	45-49	9	2.44	2.51
	50-59	27	4.55	3.14
	60-69	39	8.77	4.82

Modified from [10]

E trial results showed that tumour size, malignancy grade and nodal status are good predictors of prognosis. As is shown in Table 2 by Duffy et al. [4], the percentage of invasive cancers detected earlier was higher by diameter, nodal status and grade of malignancy when the screen-detected cancers are compared with other groups.

Figure 3 shows that survival benefit for cases detected at the prevalence or incidence screening test was maintained also after a long period of follow-up (160 months from diagnosis).

In service screening the distribution of prognostic factors in screen-detected cancers will be compared with the historical experience of the population before the start of the screening, taking into account the stage distribution of cases in non-attenders. Pathological tumour size is considered as the most relevant characteristic and should be available in most cases.

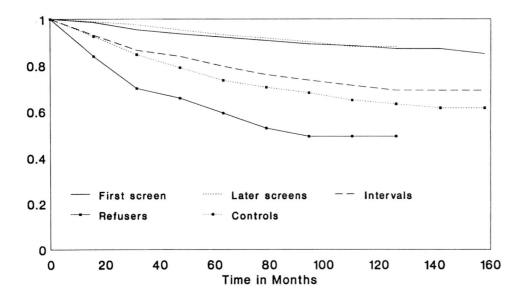

Fig. 3. Survival of women 40-69 by detection mode [2]

Table 2. Percentages of invasive cancers in categories of size, grade and node status by detection mode

Factor category	First screen	Later screens	Interval cancers	Refusals	Control group	Overall
Size						
1-9 mm	26.1	27.2	8.1	6.2	7.1	15.4
10-14 mm	29.6	26.4	21.0	8.6	15.4	21.1
15-19 mm	19.7	24.0	17.3	13.6	19.7	20.0
20-29 mm	14.1	16.5	31.5	28.4	29.0	23.7
30-49 mm	6.3	4.8	15.3	22.2	20.0	13.3
50 mm or more	4.2	1.1	6.8	21.0	8.8	6.5
Total cases	284	375	248	81	590	1578
Not known	1	1	0	0	2	4
Node status						
Negative	78.6	83.9	53.6	37.5	54.5	65.0
Positive	20.7	15.5	41.8	41.7	39.8	30.9
Distant metastases	0.7	0.6	4.6	20.8	5.7	4.1
Total cases	271	361	237	72	558	1499
Not known	14	15	11	9	34	83
Kopparberg						
Grade 1	25.2	24.2	11.5	11.1	12.6	18.2
Grade 2	37.4	52.7	34.5	40.7	42.2	42.7
Grade 3	37.4	23.1	54.0	48.1	45.2	39.1
Total cases	139	182	113	27	199	660
Not known	1	1	2	2	4	10
Ostergötland						
Grade 1	44.5	34.2	16.3	0.0	19.7	26.4
Grade 2	27.0	31.0	31.5	29.0	29.6	29.6
Grade 3	28.5	34.8	52.2	71.0	50.8	44.0
Total cases	137	155	92	31	294	709
Not known	8	35	41	21	95	203

from [4]

Interval Cancers

The definition of interval cancers depends on the schedule of the screening programme, and clinically-detected cancers should be referred to the time from the last negative test. The occurrence of interval cancers is a failure of the screening programme and is due to low sensitivity and to the compromise between the probability of incidence of new growing tumours and the costs related to a narrower interval. The shorter the interval, the greater would be the probability of detecting a new growing tumour at screening.

An increase in the proportion of screen-detected cancers is considered neither cost-effective nor practical with an interscreening interval shorter than 2 years.

Peeters et al. [12] have presented a review of interval cancer data occurring in the Nijmegen project. They classified tumours as:

1) missed cancers, when a suspect mammogram resulted from the screening test. Various reasons explained the failure of mammography and in total there were 26% of this kind of tumour;
2) radiographically occult breast cancers at the moment of diagnosis (15.7%), when cancers were not evident at the screening test and diagnosed by other techniques;
3) "true interval cancers" (58.2%) which were cancers not detectable at the screening mammogram and radiographically diagnosed during the interval.

A radiological and clinical audit of interval cancer cases is important to monitor the programme and modify the performance. They can be considered *sentinel events* and missed cancers can offer the opportunity of a revision of technical or observational errors.

An estimate of the rate of interval cancers requires a tumour registry or a pathological

Table 3. Incidence rates of breast cancer after a negative screening test, as a percentage of the incidence rates in the absence of screening (number of cases)

Study	Age group at entry into study	Time since last negative test (months)				
		0-11	12-23	24-35	36-47	48-
HIP	40-64	31.7 (41)	57.2 (27)	40.5 (5)	91.8 (7)	100 (5)
Sweden	40-49	37.8 (9)	67.6 (11)	60.0 (7)		
	50-59	11.6 (6)	29.9 (13)	46.9 (14)		
	60-69	14.3 (8)	28.1 (15)	43.1 (24)		
Utrecht	50-59	17.0 (10)	57.8 (18)	86.1 (7)	100 (10)	
	60-64	13.9 (7)	59.3 (17)	53.8 (6)	56.5 (6)	
						36-59
Florence district	40-49	24 (7)	41 (11)	98 (18)		91 (13)
	50-59	17 (6)	45 (14)	51 (10)		50 (9)
	60-69	9 (3)	17 (5)	39 (8)		55 (11)

Modified from [10]

registry collecting information of all incident cancers in the target population. Cancers in women who had a negative screening mammogram should be classified according to the date of incidence by time since the test (6 months, first and second year) and the occurrence compared with the expected incidence in the same person-year population. The occurrence of interval cancers is expressed as a proportion of the expected incidence in the absence of screening. This proportion depends on the diagnostic anticipation achieved at the previous screening test and allows one to estimate the screening test sensitivity [13]. If a subsequent screening test is not performed, the cumulative number of cases should catch up the expected number in the absence of screening (or, if available, the observed occurrence in a comparable control group). Table 3 shows the main results of the breast cancer screening studies where an analysis of the occurrence of interval cancers has been performed.

The registration of the surfacing of breast cancers after the negative test has been useful also to estimate the programme's sensitivity and mean sojourn time by modelling screening data [10,14]. Table 4 reports an estimate of programmes and it is evident, in agreement with other statistical models, that there is a certain consistency of the estimates carried out till now.

Specificity

The detection of breast cancer at the screening test depends on the sensitivity of the test. To achieve fine sensitivity, high-quality mammography should be used. At the same time screening mammography is not a diagnostic test and women will be referred for further diagnostic work-up. Referral of women who, at the end of a diagnostic work-up, will be considered as false positive causes psychological distress and financial costs to the women and society. The specificity should

Table 4. Mean sojourn time (MST), 95% confidence interval (CI) and sensitivity estimates in the Florence District Programme, Health Insurance Programme and Two County Study from interval cancer data

Age group (years)	MST (95% CI)	Sensitivity	Sensitivity (conservative)
Health Insurance Programme			
40-74	1.49 (1.13-2.18)	74	72
Two County Study			
40-49	1.18 (0.78-2.38)	69	65
50-59	4.28 (3.18-6.56)	91	90
60-69	4.01 (3.08-5.73)	88	87
Total 50-69	4.12 (3.36-5.34)	89	89
Florence District Programme			
40-44	1.34 (0.74-7.02)	72	67
45-49	2.44 (1.49-6.74)	97	89
50-54	1.63 (0.97-5.04)	88	83
55-59	5.71 (3.44-16.76)	86	84
60-64	4.68 (2.76-14.36)	91	89
65-69	6.45 (3.88-18.99)	95	94
Total 50-69	3.92 (3.01-5.82)	89	88

from [14]

be high in a programme aiming to avoid a high rate of false positives, but, at the same time, the effect of different referral policies on sensitivity must be considered. In the Great Britain National programme where single-view mammograph is suggested as screening test, 10% of referrals was considered an acceptable standard. A figure of 5% is now thought more acceptable. In the new programme started in the city of Florence in 1990 using double-view mammography, a referral rate of 4.6% has been observed (unpublished data).

With a rare disease assumption, specificity is estimated according to the following formula [15,16]:

$$\text{specificity} = \frac{\text{No. of negative screening tests}}{\text{No. SW - No. SDP patients}}$$

where SW = screened women and SDP = screen-detected patients.

Predictive Value of the Test

The positive predictive value (PV+) of the test is a measure of the test performance, estimating the proportion of women affected by breast cancer among the women referred on a suspect mammogram. The assessment of the performance of the diagnostic work-up will consider the different diagnostic procedures needed to achieve a diagnosis (ultrasonography, needle biopsy, surgical biopsy, etc.) and a PV+ of each procedure can be estimated. Criteria to assess the performance have been recently proposed by Verbeek et al [16]. In any case, a medical and radiological audit in the context of a system of quality assurance is required. Quality control of the test and of the diagnostic work-up process should be organised locally and supported by training.

Early and Final Evaluation

The evaluation of the programme in terms of mortality reduction will require several years. The registration of the date of occurrence and of the modality of detection of all cases in the target population is fundamental for future evaluation. The final evaluation can be made by comparing the expected mortality in the absence of screening with that observed, or by using a case-control approach where mortality of the screened women is compared with that of the non-attenders. This last approach might be heavily biased if the attendant population is selected on the basis of factors related to a probability of dying from breast cancer and the analysis is not adjusted [17,18].

An early evaluation of the programme is possible if the rate of the incident cases by stage is available. In the W-E trial, the analysis was carried out considering stages 0 or 1 as not advanced and cancers diagnosed at stage 2 or later as advanced. It may be that this subdivision is too approximate if the background staging in the population is good before screening (i.e., there is a high proportion of Tis or T1 in the population). In this condition, the registration system has to define the diameter of the tumours more finely, assuring a high quality of pathological reading.

Given the definition of advanced cancers, a reduction in the rate in comparison with the expected rate might be a good predictor of the programme's performance.

Table 5. Monitoring measures and the associated information requirements [3]

Measure	Qualifying comments	Additional information required	Type of evaluation provided
Compliance rate	Validation of population list	Identification of real non-compliance	Indicates potential for effectiveness of overall programme
Prevalence rate at initial screening test	Expressed as multiple of expected incidence rate in screened women	Incidence rates in non-compliance and in a comparable unscreened group, e.g. historical rates	Provide estimates of sensitivity, lead time, sojourn time and predictive value
Rate of interval cancers	Expressed as a proportion of expected incidence rate in screened women, and by time since the last screening test	Accurate identification of interval cancers, and calculation of additional incidence rates as above	
Stage (or size) distribution of screen-detected cancer	Compared to expected stage distribution in the absence of screening	Stage (or size) distribution in non-compliers and in total population before screening started	Indicates potential for reduction in absolute rate of advanced cancer
Rate of advanced cancers	Need for a definition of "advanced" which can be used for the great majority of cases given the information available. Probably based on tumour size	Stage (or tumour size) information needed historically and on cancers among non-compliers	Earlier surrogate of mortality
Breast cancer death rate	Breast cancer deaths linked to date of diagnosis		Final evaluation

Conclusions

Table 5 shows monitoring measures and associated information requirements as suggested by Day et al. [3]. The implementation of this surveillance system, together with an evaluation of the test performance in terms of specificity and positive predictive value, is a condition for the evaluation of the outcome and of the process of screening and it will be planned before starting the mammographic activity. This core of measures is a minimum set of data which should be collected at local level and supported by further information on the quality of care (for example, treatment modality). Each indicator is relevant in different phases of the screening process (first round, prevalence screening, subsequent rounds, incidence screening test, follow-up) and the early evaluation of performance indicators can allow for revision of the procedures and training through a global quality-assurance programme.

REFERENCES

1   Chamberlain J and Palli D: This monograph
2   Tabar L, Fagerberg G, Duffy SW, Day NE, Gad A, Grontoft O: Update of the Swedish Two-County program of mammographic screening for breast cancer. Radiol Clin North America 1992 (30):187-210
3   Day NE, Williams DRR, Khaw KT: Breast cancer screening programmes: the development of a monitoring and evaluation system. Br J Cancer 1989 (59):954-958
4   Duffy SW, Tabar L, Fagerberg G, Gad A, Grontoft O, South MC, Day NE: Breast screening, prognostic factors and survival-results from the Swedish Two County Study. Br J Cancer 1991 (64):1133-1138
5   Andersson I, Asperren K, Janzon L, Landerberg T, Lindholm K, Linell T, Ljungeberg O, Ranstam T, Sigfusson B: Effect of mammographic screening on breast cancer mortality in an urban population in Sweden. Results from the randomized Malmö Mammographic Screening Trial (MMST). Br Med J 1988 (297):943-948
6   Gordon RD, Venturini A, Rosselli Del Turco M, Palli D, Paci E: What healthy women think, feel and do about cancer, prevention and breast cancer screening in Italy. Eur J Cancer 1991 (27,7):913-916
7   Cockburn J, Hill D, Irwig L, De Luise T, Turnbull D, Schofield P: Development and validation of an instrument to measure satisfaction of participants at breast screening programmes. Eur J Cancer 1991 (27):827-831
8   Day NE, Walter SD: Simplified models of screening for chronic disease: estimation procedures from mass screening programmes. Biometrics 1984 (40):1-40
9   Day NE, Walter SD, Collette HJA: Statistical models of disease natural history: their use in the evaluation of screening programmes. In: Prorok PC, Miller AB (eds) Screening for Cancer. I - General Principles on Evaluation of Screening for Cancer and Screening for Lung, Bladder and Oral Cancer. UICC Technical Report Series (78), Geneva 1984 pp 55-70
10 Day NE, Walter SD, Tabar L, Fagerberg CJ, Colette HJA: The sensitivity and lead time of breast cancer screening: a comparison of the result of different studies. In: Day NE, Miller AB (eds) International Union Against Cancer Screening for Breast Cancer. Hans Huber Publishers, Toronto 1988 pp 105-109
11 Paci E, Ciatto S. Buiatti E, Cecchini S, Palli D, Rosselli Del Turco M: Early indicators of efficacy of breast cancer screening programmes: results of the Florence District Programme. Int J Cancer 1990 (46):198-202
12 Peeters PHM, Verbeek ACM, Hendriks JHCL, Holland R, Mervuriac M, Vooijs GP: The occurrence of interval cancers in the Nijmegen screening programme. Br J Cancer 1989 (59):923-932
13 Day NE: Estimating the sensitivity of a screening test. J Epidemiol Commun Health 1985 (39):364-366
14 Paci E, Duffy SW: Modelling the analysis of breast cancer screening programmes: sensitivity, lead time and predictive value in the Florence District Programme (1975-1986). Int J Epidemiol 1991 (20):852-858
15 Morrison AS: Screening in Chronic Disease. Oxford University Press, New York 1985
16 Verbeek ALM, Van den Ban MC, Hendriks JHCL: A proposal for short-term quality control in breast cancer screening. Br J Cancer 1991 (63):261-264
17 Sasco AJ, Day NE, Walter SD: Case-control studies for the evaluation in screening. J Chron Dis 1986 (39):399-405
18 Moss SM: Case-control studies of screening. Int J Epidemiol 1991 (20):1-5

Training in Mammograhic Screening

E.J. Roebuck and A.R.M. Wilson

Nottingham National Breast Screening Training Centre, City Hospital, Hucknall Road, Nottingham NG5 1PB, United Kingdom

For breast cancer screening by mammography to be effective, the processes involved must operate to the highest possible standards if the ultimate goal of reducing the mortality from breast cancer - while causing the minimum of morbidity - is to be achieved. Before embarking on any breast screening programme, the educational needs of the health-care teams to be involved must be clearly understood. It must be recognised from the outset that the mammographic screening of asymptomatic women is entirely different from the diagnostic processes involved in the assessment of symptomatic breast disease. It is very unlikely that the required expertise to undertake breast cancer screening and the management of screen-detected lesions will exist in sufficient depth and breadth within a health-care system which has not previously been involved in breast screening. It is a prerequisite of any screening programme that a comprehensive teaching programme be instituted for all the health-care professionals who will be involved in the screening process. It must also be recognised that these training programmes must be set up to provide continuing education so as to ensure that those involved are kept fully informed of all the relevant advances and changes in the field. This chapter provides a brief outline of the educational requirements of any population-based mammographic screening programme.

Who to Train and Why?

The training requirements for a successful breast screening programme are dependent upon i) which health-care professions are going to be involved in the screening process; ii) what standards of performance will be required of them and iii) what skill mix already exists amongst them.

Which Professionals Will be Involved?

There are 4 theoretical endpoints for a screening programme as defined by the limit of responsibility of the screeners (see Fig. 1). Clearly, it is in the best interest of the population being screened that a fully comprehensive, integrated screening, diagnostic and treatment service be provided, which includes specialists from all the relevant disciplines working together as a team (endpoint 4 in Fig. 1). It is recognised that many screening programmes in mainland Europe may be unable to achieve the level of service described here as the ideal. However, in the U.K., endpoint 3 is regarded as the minimum requirement and an increasing number of centres are reaping the benefits of the full comprehensive service described as endpoint 4.

There is little point in instituting a breast screening programme if the diagnostic and treatment facilities available are inadequate or unsuitable for the purposes of managing screen-detected breast lesions. In these circumstances, through no fault of its own, such a screening programme will fail. All screening programmes should be associated with fully trained multidisciplinary teams of health-care professionals with the full responsibility for providing a comprehensive service. Such a multidisciplinary team would have to include the following personnel: 1) epidemiologists;

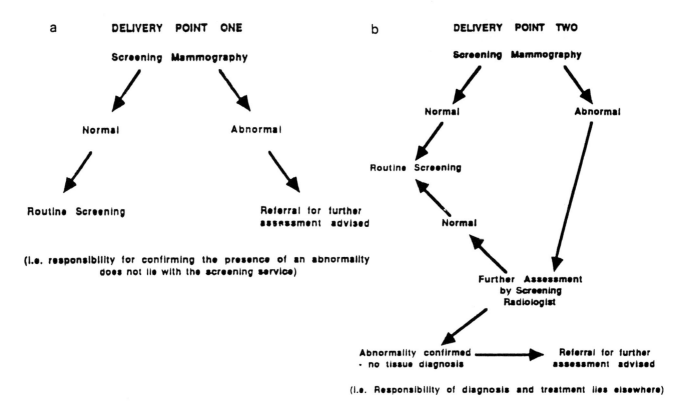

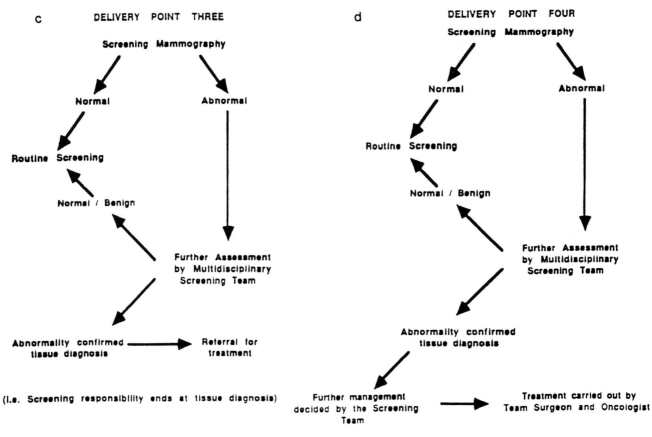

Fig. 1. Screening delivery points

2) clerical and administrative assistants; 3) service managers; 4) radiographic technicians; 5) breast care nurses; 6) radiologists; 7) surgeons; 8) pathologists; 9) oncologists.

Screening is primarily a radiological process, albeit one which requires a closer working relationship and degree of cooperation with specialists in other fields than do most of the other subspecialities of radiology. Clearly, the reading of the initial screening mammograms, in order to determine those women who require assessment or referral, and those who can be advised simply to re-attend for the next screening round, is a radiological function. It is the radiologist's responsibility to ensure that the images are of the highest quality, with a perfect balance of contrast and resolution achieved with the lowest possible dose of radiation to the breast. Basic radiological training is a vital preparation for this aspect of the service.

The basic expertise required, however, is not that of the radiologist alone. Without the professional and technical support of a highly and specifically trained radiographic technician, the standard of patient positioning will be imperfect and the control of processing parameters (which are different from those required for normal radiography) will be such that potentially good mammograms will be rendered suboptimal.

These factors alone will inevitably result in a reduction in screening sensitivity and specificity; a failure to detect breast cancers will result, leading to an unacceptably high interval cancer rate together with an unnecessarily high number of biopsies performed on women with benign disease.

It is clearly established that all screening programmes must provide training for radiographic technicians and radiologists. However, training must not be confined to these groups. Many of the lesions detected will be impalpable and surgeons and other clinicians not previously involved in screening will be unfamiliar with the specialised techniques required for the management of these types of lesion. Furthermore, in order to avoid unnecessary surgery for benign lesions and to allow for definitive preoperative treatment planning for the malignant lesions, a greatly increased number of pathologists with expertise in diagnostic breast cytology and histology will be required. Finally, the

screening programme must be subjected to scrutiny in order to assess outcomes and improve performance in areas where it is shown to be deficient. This audit requires special skills of tact in addition to simple administrative expertise and epidemiological knowledge.

It can be seen that, no matter which endpoint is considered to be the watershed of responsibility for a breast screening programme, the educational requirements of those involved in the subsequent further assessment and treatment of screen-detected lesions must be catered for besides the training provided for those directly involved in the screening process.

*Training must be targeted at **all** the healthcare workers who will be involved in managing women attending as a result of a breast screening programme.*

What Standards of Performance Are Required

If screening is not practised at the highest standards, the inevitable consequence is that the screening programme will fail to reduce breast cancer mortality in the population. Moreover, screened women will suffer unnecessarily from the problems resulting from false-negative and false-positive diagnoses with unfavourable economic consequences. Rigourous quality measures, backed by comprehensive training and quality-assurance systems, must form an integral part of the screening programme. Following screening implementation, training and quality assurance functions must be closely interrelated, the latter providing an audit of screening performance from which subsequent educational needs can be identified.

Performance standards for all aspects of a screening service must be identified and will form the basis of initial, and subsequent update, training programmes (see Table 1 for examples of performance indicators).

What Skill Mix Already Exists?

It has already been briefly mentioned, but is

Table 1. Examples of performance indicators

Category	Quality objective	Acceptable standard
BIOPSY	To maximise the positioning of marker wires in marker biopsies	> 95% should be within 10 mm of the lesion in any plane
	To minimise the time between excision and receipt of the specimen X-ray report in theatre	< 10 min 5 minutes is ideal
	To improve the operative identification of changes producing mammographic abnormalities	> 95% of impalpable lesions should be correctly identified at the first localisation biopsy
	To minimise the cosmetic disadvantage of operative biopsies carried out for diagnostic (not therapeutic) purposes	80% of biopsies which prove benign should weigh < 20 g (fresh or fixed weight)
TREATMENT	To minimise the number of repeated operations for therapeutic purposes	80% of operations carried out with a proven preoperative diagnosis of cancer should not require further operation for incomplete excision
WAITING TIMES	To minimise the interval from the basic mammogram to assessment	90% should attend an assessment centre within 1 week of the decision that further investigation is necessary and within 2 weeks of attendance for the basic mammogram
	To minimise the delay if a separate appointment has to be made for surgical assessment	< 4 days should elapse between the first recall appointment and an appointment for surgical assessment
	To minimise the interval from a surgical decision to operate for diagnostic purposes and the first offered admission date	90% should be admitted for an operative biopsy within 2 weeks of their first attendance. The surgical decision should be taken in this 2-week interval
	To minimise the interval from a surgical decision to operate for therapeutic purposes and the first offered admission date	90% should be admitted for therapeutic purposes within 2 weeks of the surgical decision to operate

worthwhile repeating, that all the skills required for successful breast screening probably do not exist in any health-care service that has no previous experience of all the processes required for mammographic screening. Even those individuals with considerable expertise and long-standing experience in the diagnosis and management of symptomatic breast problems will require further training. It cannot be over-emphasised that breast screening by mammography and the subsequent assessment and treatment of screen-detected breast abnormalities are sufficiently different from the processes of diagnosis and management of symptomatic breast disease to demand an entirely different philosophical approach.

All individuals wishing to work in, or be associated with, a screening programme, and particularly if they are to be involved in the establishment of a new programme, would benefit from training, as, indeed, will the women who entrust themselves to their care.

A multidisciplinary team of expert specialists is necessary for the provision of a total screening programme. It is unlikely that a comprehensive total programme can be established in all situations because of existing referral patterns, political, financial or other reasons. Even in these situations when a modified, subtotal screening programme is introduced, it is clearly evident that knowledge of the role of other specialists will be beneficial to every specialist upon whose practice some aspect of the screening programme impinges.

Plan of Training

For the reasons given above, training for breast screening should have a multidisciplinary base. Current practice varies from country to country and from speciality to speciality with regard to training requirements for screening. In some instances it is left entirely up to an individual to practise as he/she pleases, in others accreditation by a College or other professional body is mandatory. Specifically designed courses are available for most professions in European practice, with a content based on recommendations by the British Royal Colleges and the European Group for Breast Cancer Screening. As a consequence of the British National Breast Screening Programme, the British Breast Cancer Screening Training Centres have had

the unique opportunity to develop and establish comprehensive courses, which are now beginning to form the basic model for screening training centres throughout the world. These are based upon curricula devised by the respective Colleges and Professional Boards, with the strong influence of the European Group for Breast Cancer Screening together with individual European screening experts.

A similar National Training Programme has been developed in the Netherlands, and in Sweden periods of secondment to centres of excellence are required for radiologists. The European School of Oncology has organised courses and instituted fellowships, sponsored by The Commission of the European Communities. Specialist organisations such as The European Society of Mastology (EUSOMA) and Symposium Mammographicum organise symposia and refresher courses.

The desirability for a multidisciplinary approach to training for breast screening is becoming generally accepted, and the basic plan for every member of each professional group involved in the screening process and subsequent patient management can be expressed in an identical manner (see Table 2).

Table 2. Plan of training

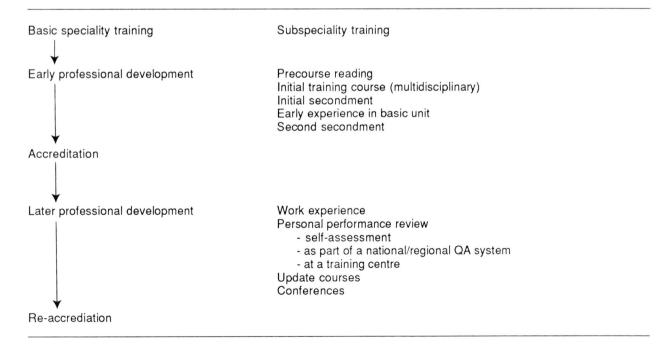

Basic speciality training	Subspeciality training
↓	
Early professional development	Precourse reading Initial training course (multidisciplinary) Initial secondment Early experience in basic unit Second secondment
↓	
Accreditation	
↓	

Later professional development	Work experience
	Personal performance review
	  - self-assessment
	  - as part of a national/regional QA system
	  - at a training centre
	Update courses
	Conferences

↓	
Re-accrediation	

The Initial Multidisciplinary Course

The object of this course is to introduce each participant to the concept of the multidisciplinary nature of breast screening and the multidisciplinary management of breast cancer patients. The course should provide an outline of the normal breast development and function, with the demonstration of radiological and immunological features of normality, normal variants and congenital anomalies. This forms the basis for consideration of benign breast conditions. Breast cancer should be dealt with in much greater depth, with the introduction of epidemiological considerations, and the variation in behaviour of different cancer types should be outlined. A comprehensive demonstration of mammographic, ultrasound, histological and cytological features should be included. Differing treatment options should be outlined with the indications and contraindications for these being explained. Following this basic introduction, the evidence for screening should be presented, with explanations of the differing results from various trials. The methods used in the critical analysis of trials should be covered during this section of the course including an explanation of the various statistical biases (lead time bias, selection bias, etc.).

Programme design is the next topic to be covered. Methods of basic screening and second-stage screening (often called assessment) should be fully discussed, with a debate on the pros and cons of the assessment process being undertaken by a dedicated multidisciplinary team as opposed to the referral of screen-detected abnormalities to a hospital for surgical assessment only. Those techniques which are by their very nature multidisciplinary should be dealt with at some depth.

The fine-needle aspiration of samples for cytology (FNAC) can be clinically performed (free hand) or achieved using ultrasound or X-ray guidance. The important points of technique of each method should be highlighted, stressing the need for good sample preparation. An explanation of how management protocols must be based upon the combined results of diagnostic cytology, imaging and clinical examination should be given.

The indications for "open" surgical biopsy should be defined, stressing the need to avoid surgical biopsy for benign conditions as much as possible. The techniques for marking of impalpable lesions prior to surgery need to be outlined, together with the surgical technique for removing the suspect lesion. This should include demonstration of the value of specimen radiography both for the surgeon at the time of operation, and subsequently for the pathologist when preparing material for histological examination.

It is also necessary to give an overview of the screening process for the woman to be screened, stressing the need to minimise anxiety, and indicating the value of trained counsellors in the screening programme.

The Specialist Theoretical Course

Having been given a multidisciplinary overview of the screening process, it is necessary for each specialist group to undergo specialist training. It is clearly impracticable to detail in this single chapter the requirements for all specialities. The Royal College of Radiologists of the United Kingdom recommended curriculum is an example (see Further Reading).

Periods of Secondment

Following the basic multidisciplinary and specialist theoretical courses, it is considered highly desirable, if not indispensable, for the budding screener of any discipline to spend a period of secondment in a functioning screening centre of proven repute. Several centres are emerging across Europe with the training expertise and screening track record, together with the facilities and time, to accommodate individuals on secondment.

The period of secondment will vary according to the speciality, and also to the degree and nature of any previous experience on the part of the trainee. For a radiologist a period of several weeks is recommended. This is best divided into 2 periods, the first, 1 or 2 weeks before the trainee commences work in his/her own basic unit, with a second period a month or two after commencing work. This second period of secondment is particularly valuable as it allows the individual trainee to discuss and solve problems identified during his/her early screening experience. Radiographers in the U.K. spend a period of one week seconded to a training centre during which time each trainee performs 50 mammograms under the supervision of a trained tutor. A month or so later, the tutor will visit the trainee in his/her own unit, and will critically examine the trainee's work, discussing and correcting problems in technique which may have become apparent. Before the trainee can be accredited as a mammographer by the College of Radiographers, the tutor must approve a further 200 mammograms taken by the trainee, as being of appropriately high quality (the quality criteria are carefully defined and are the accepted standard throughout the country).

Secondment opportunities at recognised centres of excellence must also be available to surgeons and pathologists, as well as to other groups. If it is not already the case, these professional groups should also be encouraged to be involved in the management of symptomatic breast disease.

Accreditation

It is important that, at this stage of training, accreditation for all specialist groups is promoted in order to establish acceptable standards. This will provide professional credibility and justify public confidence. Furthermore, accreditation will be of benefit from a medico-legal standpoint, and the USA experience is likely to be replicated in Europe, with insurance companies such as Blue Cross requiring accreditation as a prerequisite to reimbursement for mammography.

The details of accreditation procedures will vary from speciality to speciality, but should be harmonised throughout Europe. In the Netherlands, for example, only certified professionals may be employed in screening. For radiographers the requisite training for certification comprises a 1-week theoretical course, a 3-week practical course in positioning technique and a 3-week secondment to a recognised screening centre. The required

training for a radiologist is 2 to 3 weeks, depending upon previous experience.

It is important that each accredited individual can demonstrate that expertise is maintained, and, for this reason, periodic re-accreditation is necessary, based upon attendance at recognised courses.

Continuing Professional Development

Work Experience

To ensure that specialists acquire and maintain the necessary skills to conduct the full screening process, including assessment and the relevant aspects of patient management, it is necessary that contractual arrangements are specifically designed. The workload must be sufficiently large to enable experience and ability to be maximised. There should be adequate time allocated to the screening service, and ideally additional time to undertake symptomatic breast work. A screening service on its own cannot provide sufficient experience to achieve and maintain optimal standards amongst all the professionals involved. Moreover, it is to the mutual benefit of both symptomatic and screening services if the professionals practise in both fields.

Ultimately, performance must be judged by the achievement of outcome objectives, such as a high rate of detection of small cancers (more than 15 invasive carcinomas of 1 cm or less in diameter per 10,000 women screened), a low rate of recommendation of cases for biopsy which prove to be benign (less than 30 per 10,000 women screened) and, in the long term, a reduction in mortality from breast cancer (see Table 3 for an extended list of objectives).

It is considered that a radiologist is more likely to achieve these outcome objectives if his/her experience includes being employed for a minimum of 3, and preferably more, half days in breast imaging per week, during which a minimum of 5,000 cases are examined each year. For surgeons and pathologists, the need for symptomatic and screening experience is even greater as a result of the fewer cases referred to these specialists.

Table 3. Draft outcome objectives and standards for breast screening by mammography (November 1991)

Objective	Criteria	Acceptable standard	Achievable target
To achieve optimum quality	High contrast spatial resolution	10 line pairs per mm	12 line pairs per mm
	Minimum detectable contrast		
	5 - 6 mm	1.3	1.1
	2 mm	2.0	1.5
	1 mm	3.0	2.25
	0.5 mm	5.0	4.0
	Large area low-contrast detectability (6 mm detail)	7 details	
	Small detail contrast detectability (0.5, 0.25 detail)	7 details	
To limit radiation dose	Average glandular dose to breast using a grid	< 3 mGy per view	< 2mGy per view
To maximise the number of eligible women attending for screening	Proportion of eligible women attending	more than 70%	75%
To minimise the number of inadequate films	Number of inadequate films	< 3% of total films used	< 2%
To minimise the number of women referred unnecessarily for further tests	Referral for assessment	< 7% of women screened	4%
To minimise the number of missed cancers	In the prevalent round the proportion of cancers presenting in screened women in subsequent 12 months	< 6 in 10,000	
To maximise the number of invasive cancers detected	In the prevalent round the proportion of invasive cancers detected in women invited and screened	> 50 in 10,000 (prevalent) > 30 in 10,000 (incident)	60
To maximise the number of small invasive cancers detected	In the prevalent round the proportion of invasive cancers ≤ 10 mm in diameter (pathology measurement) detected in women invited and screened	> 15 in 10,000	> 20 in 10,000
To minimise the number of biopsies for benign disease	Benign biopsy rate	> 90 per 10,000 (prevalent) < 60 per 10,000 (incident)	50 30

Even in these circumstances it may take up to 2 years for a trained pathologist to achieve the requisite high levels of specificity in all the varied aspects of breast cytology and histology.

In addition to work experience, continuing professional development is achieved by 2 separate and distinct techniques: self-assessment, together with update courses, conferences and symposia.

Self-Assessment

Self-assessment can identify an individual's need for further training in a specific area of practice. Self-assessment is an active process of audit of one's own professional performance, including the measuring of this against the performance of one's peers. Performance indicators and guidelines have been designed for each professional group (see Table 1).

A more formal self-assessment programme has been designed for radiologists, and is being adopted by the majority of regions in the U.K. together with some centres in Australia, New Zealand and Canada. This entails a standard film set reported in the radiologist's home base, using a special report form. Results are expressed as receiver operated characteristic (ROC) curves, one for observation and one for interpretation. Each curve is displayed together with the (anonymous) curves of other radiologists. In this way an individual can judge his/her performance relative to his/her peers, and, by sequential testing, performance over time. The presence of any bias can be identified, and, when appropriate, advice on correction can be given. This tool has also been found to be valuable in the design of training programmes tailored to suit individual needs.

Update Courses

The growth of screening has been associated with the development and refining of screening techniques. It is important that training centres identify these advances in technique and organise appropriate courses to disseminate this knowledge and to instruct established screeners in new techniques and protocols. These can be 1 or 2-day courses but it is highly desirable that the course timetable allows considerable time for discussion and debate, together with the protocol demonstration where appropriate.

The Quality-Assurance System

A formal quality-assurance (QA) system is a vital element of any screening programme. The need for technical quality control is well appreciated and widely accepted with equipment testing protocols being virtually ubiquitous.

Quality assurance of professional performance has been more slowly accepted, mainly due to professional inertia. However, where QA systems have been introduced, and in the U.K. this applies to all screening units and all specialities involved in screening, it has been found that QA discussions have become an integral facet of combined training. The success of this training aspect of the professional quality-assurance system, and indeed of the whole QA system itself, results from an insistence that each profession be made responsible for its own professional QA. As a result, a "big brother" attitude has been avoided. In some areas professional jealousies are a hindrance to the adoption of a full QA system, a fact which applies to some professions more than to others.

Conferences and Seminars

An integral part of combined training is attendance at conferences and seminars which include "state-of-the-art" lectures and workshops. The importance of meeting with one's peers to discuss matters of mutual interest cannot be too highly stressed. Conferences offer an ideal opportunity for this, and, commonly, it is this aspect which contributes as much to one's continuing education as does the conference content itself.

Conclusions

1. Mammographic screening for breast cancer is different from the mammographic investigation of symptomatic disease.
2. It is unlikely that adequate experience for a breast screening programme will exist in a health care system not previously involved in screening.
3. Training for breast cancer screening is essential.
4. Training should have a multidisciplinary base so that each professional group has an awareness of the role of each of the other professional groups associated with the screening process.
5. All disciplines associated with a screening programme should receive additional training appropriate to their speciality.
6. Post-training experience should be sufficient in volume to ensure that additional experience is gained and that expertise is maintained.
7. It is to the benefit of individuals to work in both the symptomatic and screening fields, with additional benefits accruing to both screening and symptomatic services.

FURTHER READING

1   Quality Assurance Guidelines for Mammography. Prepared by a Sub-Committee of the Radiological Advisory Committee of The Chief Medical Officer of the United Kingdom (Pritchard Report). NHSBSP Publications,1987
2   Quality Assurance Guidelines for Radiologists. The Royal College of Radiologists. NHSBSP Publications, June 1990
3   Quality Assurance Guidelines for Surgeons in Breast Cancer Screening. NHSBSP Publications, May 1992
4   Guidelines for Pathologists. Prepared by a Working Party of the Royal College of Pathologists of the UK, February 1990
5   Pathology Reporting in Breast Cancer Screening. Prepared by a Working Party of the Royal College of Pathologists of the UK, February 1990
6   McLelland R, Hendrick RE, Zinninger MD, Wilcox PA: The American College of Radiology Mammographic Accreditation Programme. AJR 1991 (157):473-479
7   Gale AG: Training for mammography screening programmes. Diagnostic Imaging 1987 (9):187-193
8   Gale AG, Wilson ARM: Evaluation of radiologists' performance in reading mammograms. Br J Radiol 1991(64): 476
9   Walker GE, Gale AG, Roebuck EJ, Worthington BS: Selection and training in breast cancer screening. In: Hegarty JR and DeCann RW (eds) Psychology in Radiography II. Charge Publications 1988

Quality of Life and Breast Cancer Screening

J.C.J.M. de Haes [1,2] and H.J. de Koning [2]

1   Department of Medical Psychology, University Hospital Amsterdam and Department of Medical Decision Making,
     University of Leiden, The Netherlands
2   Department of Public Health and Social Medicine, Erasmus University Rotterdam, The Netherlands

Screening programmes have been criticised for the negative effects they have on quality of life [1]. Participation in screening would cause, in the first place, along Illich's tradition of thought, 'medicalisation'. By being confronted with too many preventive and diagnostic procedures, women would be over-concerned with health and medical issues. In the first place, their natural ways of coping with bodily inconveniences inherent in life would be impaired and thus, paradoxically, society would become less healthy. In the second place, participation in screening programmes might cause undue anxiety. This would be the case for all women participating in breast cancer screening programmes as the confrontation with the possibility of having breast cancer is frightening. It might be especially true for those women whose results are false-positive. They will have to go through an unnecessary period of diagnostic procedures, which is known to be extremely difficult.

These criticisms have to be taken seriously as the organisation of a breast cancer screening programme involves a large number of women. In the nationwide breast cancer screening programme in the Netherlands, for example, 16 million screening tests were planned in 27 years. However, the literature does not support the assumed gravity of the problem. Moreover, as will be argued, when looking at the effects of a screening programme, a more comprehensive approach must be chosen.

Several studies have been reported in the literature which belie the assumption that participation in breast cancer screening programmes will cause severe negative psycho-logical reactions. Dean and others [2] found that after 3 months, participation in screening had no effect on more than 95% of women. Ellman and others [3] found only a slight increase in worry and anxiety in the short term. Gram and co-authors [4] described serious negative reactions in some, but not in most women having a false-positive test result. These women reported to have had a difficult period, but interestingly, they said they would indeed participate again when invited for screening. We have concluded, therefore, that in the short term the negative psychological effects of screening participation are limited.

As stated, a broader point of view must also be taken. Prevention programmes may have an impact in the short term, as a result of the intervention. They are aimed, logically however, at having an effect in the long term: 1) in lowering the incidence of the disease as such in primary prevention, 2) in preventing the fatal outcome of the disease in secondary prevention, 3) in preventing the negative concomitants of disease in tertiary prevention. Thus, if one wants to investigate the effects of a prevention programme on quality of life, both short and long-term effects must be considered.

Breast cancer screening is a secondary prevention programme. The implementation of such a programme results in a shift in the stage of disease at detection and, as a consequence, in a shift in the number of women at the different stages of the disease within the population screened [5].

Figure 1 describes the shift in the number of women at different phases of the disease screening by mammography must detect small preclinical lesions and this fact further emphasises the major need for a quality-control system which will ensure both high sensitivity and specificity in the screening process. Although it is somewhat outside the scope of a single chapter on quality control in mammography, it must nevertheless be borne in mind that a fundamental item in a successful screening programme must be the establishment and maintenance of an up-to-date and accurate data-administrative system. The latter includes, as part of its data base index, information on all the women in the defined group for which results of the screening activities are registered. It is of vital importance that screening be offered to and accepted by the largest possible proportion of the population.

Equipment

The first essential element in a quality-control programme for mammography is the selection of appropriate equipment. No programme of quality-control testing with appropriate remedial action can achieve satisfactory results unless the equipment itself is of the highest possible quality. When assessing mammography equipment, the test of the image quality produced is, of course, of primary importance but there are naturally many other parameters which require to reach specification in order to make equipment acceptable. Prior to the implementation of the National Screening Programme in the United Kingdom, an attempt was made to address this particular problem by drawing up a specification for mammography equipment to be used in the programme. This specification has naturally undergone some modification since 1987 when it was first drawn up, but it represents a useful summary of the requirements for mammography equipment [3].

The other categories of equipment required for mammography are the film processing unit and the films, screens, cassettes, and daylight handling equipment. It is now widely accepted that in order to produce optimum quality mammograms, processing equipment with deep tanks and a ready means of adjustment of the overall cycle time and devel-

oper temperature are required. Experience has shown that all processors need close daily monitoring by means of a sensi-densitometry to ensure continuing optimum performance.

The choice of cassettes and daylight handling systems, and indeed processing systems themselves, may depend to some extent upon the choice of film-screen combination to be used, but it is of major importance that whichever system is chosen, it should be capable of working with films and screens of any manufacturer. This is governed by the fact that new film-screen combinations for mammography are being developed constantly and at any given moment the combination performing best in image-quality testing may be superseded by another. The selection of a film-screen combination should depend primarily upon image-quality testing with a test object or phantom which is capable of testing both resolution and low contrast discrimination. Such phantoms include the one developed by Tucker and White [4] in the late 1970s and used during the 1980s by Law and Kirkpatrick [5] for their work on film-screen combinations for mammography. More recently, the Akermann [6] and the Leeds test objects have shown improved sensitivity to varying conditions. One point which should be borne in mind is that with the film-screen combinations currently available, by far the greatest attention should be paid to image quality. None of the currently available combinations presents any serious problem in terms of the radiation dosage required to produce a satisfactory image.

The use of daylight handling equipment for mammography is now an accepted part of the state-of-the-art mammography and consistency of performance as well as a minimum of contamination of screen surfaces by dust is essential at this stage. A further important element which needs consideration is that of film-screen contact within the cassette. It was certainly the case in the past that a number of cassettes were found to be wanting in this respect even when new.

Installation of Equipment

Detailed instructions on the checking of electrical safety and installation is readily obtainable from a number of sources. The 3 European countries that currently have operational screening programmes, namely Sweden, Holland and the United Kingdom, have all developed extensive and detailed manuals for checks to be carried out upon installation of equipment, as well as the routine checks to be followed to monitor the performance of the equipment in use. On installation [7], attention must be paid to such issues as isolation and switching, protective earthing, leakage currents, fuses, trunking and cabling, cable terminations and connections, and powered ancillary equipment. It is also necessary to check the mechanical function and safety of the equipment. The first check, of course, is to ensure that the equipment is complete and properly labelled and that all mechanical and electro-mechanical functions are readily accessible. In mammography equipment the control of machine movement, locks and brakes is of prime importance, as is the checking of the compression system performance. For this purpose, there are now special test tools available and it must be ensured that the maximum compressive force does not exceed 200 Newtons [8].

The other area of major importance on acceptance is that of radiation safety, with particular attention to beam quality, collimation, interlocks and radiation leakage. Attention must naturally also be paid to the lead equivalence of the operator's protective screen. The kilovoltage delivered by the unit should be within ± 1kV of the nominal kV at at least two-thirds of the kV settings provided. Output consistency and beam quality are also assessed and, most important from the point of view of image quality, the focal spot sizes for both standard and magnification views are measured by several different techniques, namely slit camera, pinhole image of the focal spot itself, star pattern and line frequency pattern. Automatic exposure control must also be assessed at the time of installation. Finally, field uniformity and functioning of the magnification system require to be assessed on installation. Obviously a number of the checks listed at the time of acceptance of the equipment are among those checks which have to be carried out frequently during the life of the equipment. The tests to be performed and their frequency are summarised in Table 1.

Radiographic Aspects of Quality Control

A brief reference to Table 1 will reveal a number of tests which obviously fall into the province of the radiographer. The radiographer has an important role in the process of quality assurance that is specifically related to the equipment he/she uses. Those checks which relate to the working of the darkroom and its equipment, to film handling and sensitometry and the performance of cassettes and screens fall into this category. It is normally also the case that apart from checking the sensitometry on a daily basis, the other functions of the film processing equipment are controlled by the radiographer.

The primary responsibility of the radiographer in mammography is, of course, the production of the mammogram itself. This process is a demanding one, requiring a high degree of skill of the radiographer and, therefore, although not strictly part of the quality-control system, emphasis must be placed on the proper training of radiographers in the performance of the various mammographic projections. Such training should, ideally, comprise both theoretical and practical aspects and its success should be assessed against the performance of a substantial number of mammograms to required standards.

Assuming the existence of a properly trained and suitably experienced team of radiographers, the main tools in the quality control of these aspects of the process are reject analysis, self assessment and radiological assessment. The objective of reject analysis is to evaluate the quality of films produced by individual radiographers and also to establish the overall percentage of rejects on a monthly and yearly basis at individual centres. The guidelines laid down in the original Pritchard report [9] on quality assurance in mammography screening suggested that up to 3% of total rejects would be acceptable, but experience in screening programmes has shown that the norm is considerably lower. Frequently, the figure does not exceed one percent. An obvious prerequisite for a satisfactory reject analysis process is the coding of individual mammographic films with the radiographer's identity and accurate record keeping in the form of a reject analysis log. In

Table 1. Summary of tests and checks to be performed

Test title	Method	Frequency
Electrical safety of equipment and optional accessories (IPSM 3.2)		I
Equipment isolation/switching		I
Fuses*		I
Trunking & cabling*		I
Cable termination & connections		I
Panels & covers*		I
Protective earthing		I
Leakage currents		I
Electrically powered ancillary equipment*		I
Mechanical function and safety (IPSM 3.3)		I
Equipment complete	Direct	
Labelling	Direct	
Cones & collimators*	Direct	Y
Scale markings*	Direct	Y
Accessibility	Direct	Ad hoc
Movements free*	Direct	1/4Y
Locks*	Direct	1/4Y
Fail-safe devices	Direct	
Powered movement of table*	Direct	1/4Y
Adequate power*	Direct	1/4Y
Foot switches*	Direct	1/4Y
Sharp edges*	Direct Ad hoc	
Compression smooth*	Direct	M
Compression release*	Direct M	
Emergency release*	Direct	M
Max. compression	Load cell	1/2Y
Thickness indicator*	Direct 1/2Y	
Cassette insertion*	Direct Ad hoc	
AEC movement*	Direct	Ad hoc
Light adequate*	Direct	Ad hoc
Light timer*	Direct 1/4Y	
Screen markings*	Direct Ad hoc	
Screen location*	Direct Ad hoc	
Radiation safety inspection (ISPM 3.4)		***
Mains-on light*	Direct	D/Y
X-rays-on light*	Direct D/Y	
Total filtration	HVT/Direct	1/2Y
Filter interlock	Direct	1/2Y
Diaphragm interlock	Direct	1/2Y
Exposure termination	Direct	1/2Y
Exposure control position	Direct	I
Exposure control design	Direct	I
Exposure control function	Direct	I
Entrance light*	Direct	W
Lead equivalence marking	Direct	I

Table 1. Summary of tests and checks to be performed (cont.)

Test title	Method	Frequency
Screen gap	Direct	I
Visibility etc.*	Direct	I
Leakage	Ion ch	Y
Screen trans	?	I
Film/table edge	?	I
X-ray/film	Film	I
X-ray light	Film	Y

X-ray tube characteristics (IPSM 3.5)

Tube kV	kVmeter 1/2Y	
Output consistency	Ion ch	1/2Y
HVT/filtration	A1	1/2Y
Focus size	Slit etc	1/2Y

Automatic exposure control (IPSM 3.5)

Consistency	Ion ch	Y
Sensor area	Ion ch	Y
Thickness	Slabs	W
kV	Slabs	1/4Y
Other factors	Ion ch	1/4Y
Density control	Ion ch	1/4Y
Guard timer	Lead	Y

Other features of X-ray sets (IPSM 3.5)

Field uniformity	Film/D	Y
Magnification	Film	I/Mod
Grid	Film/ion	I/Mod

Dark room

Light tight	Direct	Ad hoc
Safelights	Direct 1/2Y	
Temperature	Direct	1/2Y

Processor and chemicals

APU temperature	Therm.	W
APU speed	Watch	1/4Y
Replenishment	?	M
Sp. gravit/pH	?	M
Residual hypo	?	M
Sensitometry	S.D.	D

Cassettes, screens & film

Cassette/screens ID	Direct	Ad hoc
Screen film contact	Test tool	1/2Y
Light tightness	Direct	I/Ad hoc

Table 1. Summary of tests and checks to be performed (cont.)

Test title	Method	Frequency
Relative screen sensitivity	Slabs	I/Ad hoc
Cassette/screen cleaning	?	D
Stock control	Direct	W
AEC	Blocks	D/W/M
Illuminators & viewing room		
Visual check	Direct	W
Illumination	Photom	1/2Y
Ambient light	Photom	1/2Y
Breast dose		
Rapid check	Calc.	1/2Y
Rapid check	Calc.	1/2Y
Full dose	Ma & ion	1/2Y
Reporting	Direct	1/2Y
Image quality		
Daily check	Simple phantom	D
Weekly/monthly check	Compl. phantom	W/M

Key to test frequencies: D = daily; W = weekly; M = monthly; 1/4Y = 3-montly; 1/2Y = 6-monthly; Y=yearly; I = at initial acceptance testing and again at end of warranty; Mod. = at initital acceptance testing and again at end of warranty and also whenever any relevant modification is made to the equipment

*　　should also be checked by the user by simple visual inspection at monthly intervals thereafter and the results recorded

***　acceptance testing, then as started

the log, the reason for the rejection of a film and its repetition are carefully recorded and Table 2 lists examples of such codings [7]. In the 'A' section of Table 2, the errors are attributable to the radiographer, whereas in section 'B' the fault is a mechanical one of some type.

A carefully maintained reject analysis log book kept by the radiographer who enters the date, film identification number, reject code, side(s) affected by the fault(s) and the radiographer's code number will enable continuous improvement to professional standards.

The maintenance of high morale and interest in the production of the highest possible quality of mammograms is fundamental to the quality control system. Individual self-assessment is an essential part of this process which should be continuous with each radiographer checking her/his own films as they are processed and coding all rejects according to the codes indicated in Table 2.

The final decision as to the acceptability of film quality has to be taken by the radiologist, and this will normally be done at the time of reporting. The radiologist is ultimately responsible for the quality of the films produced and films rejected by the radiologist should again be logged in a similar way to those rejected by the radiographer at an early stage. It should be noted that in centres carrying out large numbers of examinations the use of computer technology to record and analyse the data is worthwhile.

Table 2. Reject analysis coding

A. Radiographer's faults	B. Machine faults
Inaccurate positioning	Film fogging
Double exposure	Processor malfunction
Movement unsharpness	Emulsion fault
Underexposure/overexposure	X-ray unit malfunction
Extraneous objects	Cassette fault
Cassette wrong way around	
Film wrong way around	

Assessment of Radiation Dose

The constant monitoring of the radiation dose produced by mammographic examination is an important element in any mammography unit, but it is of particular importance in a screening programme when healthy women are being irradiated for no other reason than that of screening. On a day-to-day basis, this aspect of quality control is also, to a great extent, the responsibility of the radiographer. Obviously, such methods of dosimetry as direct measurement by thermoluminescent dose meters or other direct methods of dosimetry are the responsibility of the physicist, but on a day-to-day basis the radiographer can record, and should record, the mAS and the compressed breast thickness in specified numbers of patients. This process can, by calculation, give an indirect measure of breast dosage received.

Reporting of the dose measurements must be carried out in such a way that action can be taken if agreed norms are exceeded.

Assessment of Radiation Quality

The continual monitoring of the image quality produced by the mammographic system is, of course, central to the maintenance of the quality of the programme. The radiographer should on a daily basis take a radiograph of a simple test object as a rough check to verify the system. This particular film should be taken in standard conditions on each occasion and the resulting films must be inspected immediately so that any problem that becomes evident can be dealt with immediately. In addition to the daily image, quality check films should be taken of a more complex and more sensitive test object on a weekly, or a monthly basis, so as to ensure that a more subtle degradation of image quality is not taking place. In this instance, films are usually taken both in standard conditions and with magnification. It is interesting to note that past experience in screening programmes has shown that this latter procedure can detect early and subtle deteriorations in various aspects of the image production chain as a result of a gradual change in image scores over a period of some months.

Radiological Aspects of Quality Control

Generally, the individual with overall responsibility for the outcome of the screening programme is the radiologist. Normally, the responsibility for implementing, evaluating and updating the quality-control programme will also rest with the radiologist in charge of the screening programme. Obviously, the radiologist places considerable reliance on the radiographers and physicists working in the screening team, for those aspects of quality control and quality assurance systems already discussed. However, the radiologist is the individual wholly responsible for the reading and interpretation of the mammograms, and for action taken on the identified abnormal results.

Training

It is fundamental to the success of a screening programme, or indeed a symptomatic mammography programme, that any radiologist involved in it should be adequately trained to the task in hand. The basic requirement of a radiologist reading screening mammograms is of course the ability to detect the subtle abnormalities which may indicate the presence of cancer. This can only be acquired on the basis of appropriate theoretical teaching allied to practical demonstration and teaching, backed up by a considerable amount of film-reading experience. Experience gained in various screening programmes has indicated that there is an important learning curve for radiologists involved in this particular activity extending over a range of 6-18 months, depending on the level of activity and on the radiologist's age and aptitude.

It must also be remembered that sufficient ongoing experience is necessary to maintain expertise once it has been initially acquired. The recommendations of the Pritchard report [9] in the United Kingdom, for instance, specify that in order to continue to be sufficiently experienced to read screening mammograms, the radiologist must read at least 5,000 sets of screening mammograms per year, and while this is only an estimate of what is required for the maintenance of expertise, there is little doubt that the figure is of the correct order. Naturally, however, the training and experience to enable the radiologist to read the mammograms is only a part of the responsibilities. The radiologist must also be trained and experienced in the process of assessing screen-detected abnormalities, in the application and interpretation of other mammographic techniques, in ultrasound imaging of the breast and in the techniques of ultrasound-guided and stereotaxically-guided fine-needle aspiration of impalpable breast lesions. The latter naturally includes experience in the marking of lesions for surgical biopsy. Furthermore, the radiologist must have extensive practical knowledge of the technical aspects of mammogram production and of the correct methodology of positioning for mammography, so that guidance can be given to other members of the screening team.

Performance Indicators

While it is relatively straightforward to assess the performance of the system producing the mammographic image, monitoring the performance of the interpretation of the image is less easy and requires certain key data. The fundamental statistic above all others by which a radiologist judges his/her performance is obviously the number of cancers that have occurred between screening episodes - possibly including some which have been missed for a variety of reasons. This is the so-called interval cancer rate and is a figure which, in many countries, is in fact very difficult to estimate. Day [10] has estimated that there should be no more than 25% of the expected incidence of breast cancer in the first 2 years after a negative mammogram, and no more than 60% of the expected incidence in the third year after a negative mammogram. This can be regarded as a very good guide to the sort of level of interval cancers to be expected. Other performance indicators are in varying degrees more readily accessible, however, than the interval cancer rate. The first which becomes available in a screening programme is the recall rate. This is the rate at which initial screening mammograms are reported as abnormal, or as requiring further evaluation. Recommendations as to the appropriate level for recall vary. The initial rate recommended in the United Kingdom in the Pritchard report [9] was 10%, but subsequent experience in the U.K. Screening Programme has shown that figures nearer to 5% are more frequent, and this is certainly confirmed by the Swedish and the Dutch experience where 5% or less is commonplace. The question of dual reading of screening mammograms has a very definite bearing on the likely recall rate. There can be little question that dual reading of screening mammograms by experienced radiologists increases the sensitivity of the test but if mammograms are read independently and all positive calls acted upon, then there clearly is a risk of an increase in the overall recall rate. Practical experience in a number of screening programmes has shown, however, that this problem is largely confined to the early months of a programme, when the radiologists are themselves in a learning phase [11].

The crude cancer detection rate is a basic measure of the success of a screening programme. Clearly, the crude cancer detection rate depends fundamentally upon the natural incidence of breast cancer in any given area, and Day [10] has again calculated that the crude cancer detection rate in the first screening round should be no less than 3 times the underlying incidence rate. This translates, for example in the United Kingdom, in Sweden or in Holland, to a rate which should exceed 5 cancers per thousand women screened in the 50-65 age group. A refinement of the crude cancer detection rate which was developed by Price and utilised in the Pritchard report [9] in the U.K. has been the detection rate for small invasive cancers. In the U.K. setting, the calculated rate in the first screening round is that 1.5 invasive carcinomas of less than 1 cm in diameter should be detected per thousand women screened. Translating this figure into a relationship with the natural incidence rate results in an approximate equation with the natural incidence rate.

The positive predictive value of the screening test and the subsequent work-up to the point of open surgical biopsy should be in the order of 40% in the initial screening round and should increase in following screening rounds with 50% or better, as a target. In other words, the malignant to benign ratios for open surgical biopsy should achieve the rate of 1:1. It must be added that this not very ambitious target has already been equalled and, in many instances, has been exceeded by many screening programmes now in existence. Several other measurable parameters of performance have been suggested by Day et al. [10] as being indicative of the efficiency of the performance of a screening programme and a number of these relate to stage distribution. It is suggested that no more than 40% of the cases should be at stage II or more advanced at the first screening round, and that figure should drop to no more than 30% in subsequent rounds. The reduction in the rate of advanced cancer should not be less than 30% in the target population 7 years after the first invitation has been sent. The final measure, which will be very late in appearing, is of course the ultimate measure of the success, or otherwise, of a screening programme, and that is the reduction in the mortality rate which should exceed 25% in the target population free from breast cancer when the first invitation was sent. This measure is taken 10 years after the start of a programme.

Programme Organisation

In many instances the radiologist will be responsible for the overall performance of the programme and will therefore also be responsible for monitoring and recording of other items in the programme such as 1) number of women invited; 2) number of women screened; 3) number of women recalled for technical reasons; 4) time interval between invitation to screening and referral to assessment; 5) type and number of additional tests performed; 6) number of fine-needle aspiration cytology examinations performed; 7) number of needle localisation biopsies performed; 8) number of stereotaxic or ultrasound-guided fine needle-aspiration cytologies performed; 9) number of women managed by early follow-up.

Dual Reading

Reference to the desirability of dual reading of screening mammograms has already been made, and when this procedure is carried out it is possible to calculate the performance of each radiologist. This clearly is a sensitive matter and the results of such assessments must remain confidential within the profession. There is little doubt, however, that recourse to dual reading increases the sensitivity of the test by a factor which may be as high as 20% in the early stages of a programme. In the first 12 months' running of the South East Scotland screening programme, for example, no less than 22% of the cancers detected were not observed by one of the two film readers. This rate fell sharply over succeeding years as newly trained readers gained experience, but from the experience gained in many centres it is clear that an increase in sensitivity will always be obtained by dual reading, probably of the order of 5-10% of cancers detected.

Review of Quality-Control Data

Due to the recording of the considerable amount of quality-control information, data should be reviewed on a regular basis to assess the performance of the screening programme. In addition, the radiologist involved in screening programmes should review in detail films of interval cancer patients, the films of all particularly early cancers, and films of those cancers which have been missed by one or more of the film readers who have seen the films. Experience has shown that the latter group, as would be expected, contains valuable teaching material demonstrating very early subtle changes.

In conclusion, it can be said that the processes involved in adequate comprehensive quality control of mammography screening programmes are extensive, wide ranging and complex. However, with a screening test such as mammography, particular attention to the entire process of quality control in the production and interpretation of the mammographic image is the only sure route to success.

REFERENCES

1   Muir Gray JA: General Principles of Quality Assurance in Breast Cancer Screening. Screening Publications. National Breast Cancer Screening Education Programme, March 1990
2   Peeters P: Proceedings 15th Anniversary of Nijmegen Breast Screening Programme. September 1990
3   Guidance notes for health authorities on mammographic equipment requirements for breast cancer screening. STD/1987/34. DHSS
4   White DR, Tucker AK: A test object for assessing image quality in mammography. Br J Radiol 1980 (53):331-335
5   Kirkpatrick AE, Law J: A comparative study of films and screens for mammography. Br J Radiol 1987 (60):73-78
6   Law J: A new phantom for mammography. Br J Radiol 1991 (64):116-120
7   Quality Assurance Manual. Scottish Breast Screening Service. Scottish Quality Assurance Reference Centre, Scottish Office, March 1990
8   DHSS 1987/34 para1.4.8
9   Quality assurance guidelines for mammography. Report prepared by a working group under the chairmanship of Dr. John Pritchard for the radiological advisory committee of the chief medical officer (England), 1988
10   Day NE, Williams DDR, Khaw KT: Breast cancer screening programmes: The development of a monitoring and evaluation system. Br J Cancer 1989 (59):954-958
11   Proceedings of radiology quality assurance group. National Health Service Breast Screening Programme 1991

Quality Control in Mammography

Alistair E. Kirkpatrick

Scottish Health Service, South East Scotland Breast Screening Programme, Breast Screening Centre, 26 Ardmillan Terrace, Edinburgh EH11 2JL, Scotland

In those countries that have acquired considerable experience in the field of breast cancer screening by mammography, it is now generally acknowledged that a comprehensive system of quality assurance is a fundamental requirement. The reason for this is that mammography is a far from ideal screening test in that it requires a very high level of performance in the production and interpretation of the images to perform the function of a screening test successfully. In this context it is perhaps relevant to contrast mammography with a simple chest X-ray as a screening test. To produce a satisfactory chest X-ray, any standard films with moderate performance can be used: the performance of the intensifying screens is likewise uncritical, there is no need for a moving grid, exposure control is simple with considerable latitude, and the equipment required to produce the image can be very basic. There are no particular problems when processing the exposed film and the variations in normal appearances are considerably less than is the case in mammography. A satisfactory screening mammogram, on the other hand, requires a very high quality dedicated film-screen combination whose performance needs constant checking. The mammography unit required to produce the mammogram is necessarily dedicated and is subject to a detailed high specification in all aspects of its operation which again need constant monitoring. Positioning of the patient for the examination is a highly skilled operation and requires considerable training and experience. The processing of mammograms is a specialised process and dedicated processing facilities are needed. As with all other aspects of image production, the performance of the processing unit should be closely monitored. Sensitometric testing of the processor is necessary daily and sometimes more frequently. Finally, a high level of training and experience is needed to enable a radiologist to read screening mammograms successfully and reliably. For the process of screening by mammography to be successful, all elements in the chain must operate at an optimal level or the number of cancers missed by the process inevitably rises. Thus, mammography can only be an efficient screening test if strict quality-assurance guidelines exist for all aspects of any screening programme.

It is worth now considering in more detail the terms *quality assurance* and *quality control*. Gray [1] has defined the process of quality assurance as (1) the continual pursuit of excellence and (2) as a secondary feature, the maintenance of minimum standards. Quality assurance is achieved by the application of a quality-control programme - a series of tests and performance indicators which are applied to each element in the production and interpretation of the mammographic image. In spite of the technical problems in achieving and maintaining satisfactory standards, breast cancer screening by means of mammography has been shown to reduce the mortality from the disease and present estimates suggest that, given a 100% compliance rate in the population invited for screening, the mortality reduction would be of the order of 40%. A corresponding fall-off in the mortality rate reduction is naturally anticipated with lesser degrees of compliance, a 70% compliance would result in 28% reduction in mortality and a 60% compliance would result in approximately 18% reduction in mortality [2]. In order to achieve its aim,

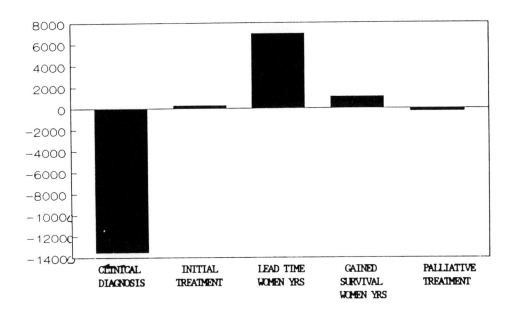

Fig. 1. The simulated shift in the number of women in different phases in the year 2000 in the Netherlands as a result of the nationwide breast cancer screening programme

process in the Netherlands in the year 2000. It is interesting to note that fewer women will undergo clinical diagnosis as the number of self-referrals and referrals by primary physicians will decrease. Due to the increase in screen-detected cancers, more women will undergo primary treatment. The number of lead-time women-years is given: some women will live with the disease, while the disease would not have been diagnosed at this stage without the screening programme. Gained survival is the survival of those women who would otherwise have died as a result of the disease, but do survive through earlier detection. Finally, palliative treatment is less frequent as a higher proportion of women with breast cancer will be cured. When investigating the impact of the screening programme, all these effects have to be taken into account. This was done in the report of the Forrest Committee [6], but in a rather simplified way: one quality of life value was given for all stages of the disease. In the Dutch cost-effectiveness analysis a more elaborate approach was chosen. The different phases of the disease process were described on the basis of the literature; these phases were evaluated by public health and breast cancer experts and the values were inserted in the cost-effectiveness analysis. Thus, a quality-of-life adjustment of the cost-effectiveness of the programme could be established [7,8].

Value Given to Screening, Disease and Treatment Phases

The stages considered relevant in the quality-adjusted effectiveness analysis were the following: screening participation, diagnosis, surgery, radiotherapy, chemotherapy and hormonal therapy in initial treatment, disease-free periods up to and after one year (after mastectomy and breast-conserving therapy), palliative treatment modalities and terminal illness.

Empirical investigation of quality of life in all these phases would be too extensive a project. Therefore, the descriptions were derived from the aggregation of data from the literature. A medline search into the literature up to 1989 resulted in 252 articles. Of these, 176 dealt with the impact of the different phases of the disease process on the quality of life of breast cancer patients.

As can be seen in Table 1, most of these articles related to initial treatment and the disease-free periods. Few empirical studies concerned palliative treatment and terminal illness in particular. Physical and emotional effects were described in most studies while many referred to the social effects of the disease. A global evaluation of the situation integrating specific aspects was given in a limited number of studies only. A utility score was reported in one paper only.

Table 1. Content of papers dealing with quality of life and breast cancer (screening)

	Total (N=176)	Empirical (N=139)
Screening attendance	6	3
Diagnostic phase	25	13
Initial surgery	47	30
Initial chemotherapy	31	22
Initial radiotherapy	13	3
Initial hormonal therapy	7	5
Breast reconstruction	15	11
Disease free 3 months - 1 year after mastectomy	47	38
> 1 year after mastectomy	55	46
3 months - 1 year after breast-conserving therapy	10	8
> 1 year after breast-conserving therapy	17	12
Palliative treatment + surgery	11	8
+ chemotherapy	33	30
+ hormonal therapy	19	17
+ radiotherapy	10	8
Terminal illness	5	2
General	8	4
Physical	132	104
Psychological	117	93
Social	67	49
Global	11	11
Utility	2	1

As the aggregation of specific data on the physical, psychological and social concomitants of disease in a global evaluation for the different disease and treatment phases was rarely given, a valuation of these phases had to be obtained empirically. Therefore, the specific data were first summarised for every disease and treatment phase and a description was made on the basis of these summaries. Subsequently, experts in public health and breast cancer epidemiology or treatment (N=31) were asked to award scores to the descriptions of the different stages. Twenty-seven of them responded. The scores were marked on a visual analogue scale, ranging from 0 to 100. Thus, median assessment scores could be calculated and transformed into the so-called utility scores, as suggested by Torrance [9]. A utility score incorporates the assessment of a health/disease state and the willingness to trade off length of life against the loss in quality of life in that state. By subtracting the utilities found from 1.00, a loss in utility is calculated. These scores were necessary to insert quality of life in the cost-effectiveness model.

In Table 2 the median evaluations and corresponding utilities are given for the different disease and treatment phases. The screening-participation period was scored most favourably by respondents, much higher evaluations than any other phase. Disease-free periods were given higher scores than any treatment or diagnostic phase. As expected, patients undergoing breast-conserving therapy were considered "better off" than those having undergone a mastectomy. The diagnostic phase was considered burdensome, but not as much as the treatment phases. Chemotherapy was looked upon as the most intrusive treatment modality while surgery alone was considered the least bur-

Table 2. Median valuations and corresponding utilities of the diagnostic/disease/treatment phases*

		Median	Utility	Loss in utility (1-u)
1.	Terminal illness	17	.288	.712
2.	Palliative + chemotherapy	34	.531	.469
3.	Palliative + radiotherapy	38	.591	.419
4.	Palliative + surgery	41	.617	.383
5.	Palliative + hormonal therapy	45	.663	.337
6.	Initial chemotherapy	50	.717	.283
7.	Initial radiotherapy	59	.803	.197
8.	Initial hormonal therapy	61	.820	.180
9.	2 months - 1 year after mastectomy	64	.844	.156
10.	Initial surgery	67	.867	.133
11.	Diagnostic phase	71	.895	.105
12.	2 months - 1 year after breast-conserving therapy	74	.914	.086
13.	Disease free > 1 year after mastectomy	80	.947	.053
14.	Disease free > 1 year after breast-conserving therapy	83	.960	.040
15.	Screening attendance	94	.994	.006

*   the order is according to the utility given

densome type of treatment. Quality of life was scored lower in palliative treatment phases than in initial treatment phases. Again, chemotherapy was considered most burdensome. Finally, the terminal illness phase was considered synonymous with the lowest quality of life.

Quality Adjustment in the Effectiveness Analysis

Given the different screening, disease and treatment phases and their valuation, one can compute a quality-adjustment factor if the duration of these phases is given. This duration was established on the basis of clinical work and chart reviews (see Table 3) [7]. Data from Dutch and Swedish screening trials about the course of the disease after screening have been used to predict the number of women in the different phases with and without a screening programme [8,10]. Quality adjustment can be computed by multiplying the number of women in the stage by the score and the duration of that phase.

Quality-adjusted life years = sum (over phases) of utility x duration x number of women.

The same can be done for the situation with and without screening. By subtracting both, the effect of the programme on quality-adjusted life years is given.

In Table 3 the correction for quality of life for every disease/treatment phase is given separately first. As can be seen in the terminal illness phase and in palliative treatment modalities, a positive effect of the screening programme is expected. This is especially true for chemotherapy and hormonal therapy. A substantial positive effect is also expected as a result of the smaller number of women receiving initial hormonal therapy. The number of women having to undergo a mastectomy will decrease after screening because of earlier detection. Therefore, a positive effect is expected in the first year after diagnosis.

On the other hand, a number of negative effects is predicted, e.g., an increase in the number of women undergoing breast-conserving therapies and in the number of women-years after mastectomy. This is the so-called lead-time effect. Some more

Table 3. Number of women, multiplied by the duration of states (women-years), in the situation with or without breast cancer screening and the correction as a result of quality adjusting the effect

		Duration	Number of women		Quality adjustment
			with screening	without screening	
1.	Terminal illness	1 month	271,815	288,862	1,008
2.	Palliative + chemotherapy	4 months	271,815	288,862	2,665
3.	Palliative + radiotherapy	1 month	271,815	288,862	593
4.	Palliative + surgery	5 weeks	271,815	288,862	666
5.	Palliative + hormonal therapy	14 months	271,815	288,862	6,700
6.	Initial chemotherapy	6 months	31,934	31,934	0
7.	Initial radiotherapy	2 months	388,937	378,634	- 340
8.	Initial surgery	2 months	580,847	571,620	- 205
9.	Initial hormonal therapy	2 years	188,742	198,313	3,449
10.	2 months - 1 year after mastectomy	10 months	309,271	320,188	1,416
11.	Diagnostic phase	5 weeks	1,244,643	1,257,049	125
12.	2 months after breast-cons. therapy	10 months	255,687	234,521	- 1,519
13.	Disease free > 1 year after mastect.	life expectancy	3,203,247	3,169,573	- 1,800
14.	Disease free > 1 year after conservative therapy	life expectancy	3,372,980	2,907,354	- 18,512
15.	Screening attendance	1 week	15,768,572	0	- 1,790
	Correction for double counting				- 686
	Total correction for quality of life				- 8,230
	Effect breast cancer screening on life-years gained				259,704
	Effect breast cancer screening on quality-adjusted life-years gained				251,474

women will have to undergo initial surgery and radiotherapy. Finally, the women participating in screening experience a slight negative effect. This effect has been assessed as only somewhat negative by the experts and, moreover, relates to a very short period. This effect, therefore, does not have an important impact on the quality adjustment in the screening effectiveness analysis.

Conclusion

Considering all these effects together, as can be seen from Table 3, the difference between the situation with and without screening is computed to be 259,704 woman-years in the Netherlands. This result, which is considered a substantial gain, is based on a 27-year screening programme organised for women between 50 and 70 years of age at 2-year intervals. If this effect is adjusted for quality of life, breast cancer screening leads to a gain of 251,474 woman-years. Taking quality of life into account, the difference with and without screening is small: 3.2%. We did, therefore, conclude in our earlier paper that the issue of quality of life is not substantial enough in breast cancer screening to refrain from organising such programmes [7].

A number of variants have been computed to establish the firmness of this conclusion.

Instead of the median, the mean scores have been inserted into the model. Also, a discounting of 5% for future effects was proposed. Finally, on the basis of the range in the given scores, "favourable" and "unfavourable" variants were taken. In the most negative case, the quality of life adjustment on the analysis of effectiveness made a difference of -19.7%. In the most positive one the adjustment was +3.2%. We therefore concluded that the "true" adjustment must be somewhere in between, about 8% loss in effectiveness. This figure still leads to the conclusion that quality of life is not the main consideration when deciding on a breast cancer screening programme.

Some further studies are needed. The data derived from the literature are stronger for some phases than for others. It was noted that little empirical work was reported about the palliative treatment phases and especially about terminal illness. More thorough findings on these phases would be necessary. Also, the scores provided by patients or by the general public might have led to dissimilar conclusions. The method used here was not yet suitable for lay people. The description of the state of health had to be complex on the one hand so as to cover the domains described properly, but on the other hand, a more simple description might facilitate an approach by broader populations.

Ideally, one would want a large prospective longitudinal study, following up patients and non-patients from screening onwards. Given the present results, however, the conclusion that quality of life is not a major negative factor as a result of positive long-term effects must be taken as a starting point.

REFERENCES

1 Roberts MM: Breast screening: time for a rethink? Br Med J 1989 (299):1153-1155
2 Dean C, Roberts MM, French K, Robinson S: Psychiatric morbidity after screening for breast cancer. J Epidemiol Comm Hlth 1986 (42):1239-1241
3 Ellman R, Angeli N, Christians A, Moss S, Chamberlain J, Maguire P: Psychiatric morbidity associated with screening for breast cancer. Br J Cancer 1989 (60):781-784
4 Gram IT, Lund E, Slenker SE: Quality of life following a false positive mammogram. Br J Cancer 1990 (62):1018-1022
5 de Koning HJ, van Oortmarssen GJ, van Ineveld BM, van der Maas PJ: Breast cancer screening: its impact on clinical medicine. Br J Cancer 1990 (61):292-297
6 Forrest P: Breast Cancer Screening. Report to the Health Ministers of England, Wales, Scotland and Northern Ireland by a working group chaired by Prof. Sir Patrick Forrest. London 1986
7 de Haes JCJM , de Koning HJ, van Oortmarssen GJ, van Agt HME, de Bruyn AE, van der Maas PJ: The impact of a breast cancer screening programme on quality-adjusted life-years. Int J Cancer 1991 (49):538-544
8 de Koning HJ, van Ineveld BM, van Oortmarssen GJ, de Haes JCJM, Collette HJA, Hendriks JHCL, van der Maas PJ: Breast cancer screening and cost-effectiveness; policy alternatives, quality of life considerations and the possible impact of uncertain factors. Int J Cancer 1991 (49):531-537
9 Torrance GW: Social preferences for health states: an empirical evaluation of three measurement techniques. Socio-Econ Plan Sci 1976 (10):129-136
10 van Oortmarssen GJ, Habbema JDF, van der Maas PJ , de Koning HJ, Colette HJA, Verbeek ALM, Geerts AT, Lubbe KTN: A model for breast cancer screening. Cancer 1990 (66): 1601-1612